# ALONE IN THE CROWD
## Living Well with Endometriosis

Endometriosis Survivor
Author | Speaker | Psychologist
Founder EndoPositive International™

Let's connect at
www.AniaLive.com
and www.EndoPositive.org

*Ania G*

Call me once you are done reading my book.
I want to hear from you!

773.456.6166

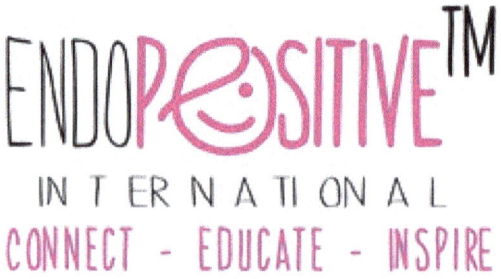

Follow EndoPositive International™
## EndoPositive.org

Empowering the 175 million women globally who suffer from Endometriosis, giving them a stage - giving them a voice

For real-time events, book signings & my latest recipes from my healthy and delicious kitchen. I would love tomeet you and hear your story. Connect with me Online, I want to hear from and will follow you back:

Twitter.com/AniaWrites
Instagram.com/AniaWrites
Linkedin.com/EndometriosisAuthorAniaG
Facebook.com/AuthorAniaG
Pinterest.com/AuthorAniaG
AniaLive.com

# ALONE IN THE CROWD

## LIVING WELL WITH ENDOMETRIOSIS

By Ania G

Published by

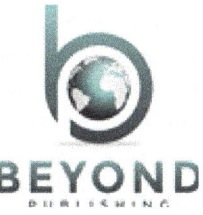

New York • Dallas • Los Angeles • Sydney
Copyright © 2015 by Ania G

# ALL RIGHTS RESERVED

No part of this publication may be reproduced, distributed, or transmitted in any form or by any means, including photocopying, recording, or other electronic or mechanical methods, without the prior written permission of the publisher, except in the case of brief quotations embodied in critical reviews and certain other noncommercial uses permitted by copyright law. For permission requests, write to the publisher, addressed "Attention: Permissions Coordinator,"

info@beyondpublishing.net

Orders by U.S. trade bookstores and wholesalers.
Please contact BeyondPublishing.net
First Edition Beyond Publishing soft cover edition June 2015

In the text that follows, some people's names and identifying characteristics have been changed.

The Beyond Publishing Speakers Bureau can bring authors to your live event. For more information or to book an event contact the Beyond Publishing Speakers Bureau at speak@BeyondPublishing.net

For all the good stuff go to www.AniaLive.com and www.EndoPositive.org
Manufactured and printed in the United States of America

10 9 8 7 6 5 4 3 2 1
Library of Congress Cataloging-in-Publication Data has been applied for.
ISBN 978-0-9961486-2-7
ISBN 978-0-9961486-3-4 (ebook)

# Contents

Foreword
Words from the Author
Prologue..................................................................13
Chapter 1: Coming to America............................19
Chapter 2: Facing the Enemy..............................40
Chapter 3: What is Endometriosis?.....................58
Chapter 4: Misconceptions and Myths................65
Chapter 5: Fertility Issues....................................80
Chapter 6: What is a Woman?.............................88
Chapter 7: Dealing with Pain...............................97
Chapter 8: Men and Women..............................111
Chapter 9: Secret Suffering...............................126
Chapter 10: Deciding on Treatment...................129
Chapter 11: Life with Endometriosis..................140
Chapter 12: EndoPositive International™...........147
Appendix I: Trauma............................................152
Appendix II: Conventional Treatment.................154
Appendix III: Alternative Treatments..................155
Appendix IV: Eating with Endo..........................156
Appendix V: The Sweet Life...............................160
Appendix VI: The Juicy Life................................163

# Foreword

It is my great pleasure to hand you over Ania Gurynowicz's book Alone in the Crowd.

We live in the times of the greatest global health crisis and at the same time growing health awareness among the general population, especially in developed countries. As a graduate of NY based Institute for Integrative Nutrition (IIN), the largest holistic nutrition school in the world, I see by the growing number of students from all over the world, mostly of whom are women, the burning desire to fix the current modern ailments by going back to the traditional, non-invasive healing methods which include finding out the root cause, taking out what doesn't serve the body, replacing it with something good, nutritious and positive.

Alone in the Crowd matches perfectly that desire. It is a reflection of the modern day woman, her journey through life, emotions, desires, hopes, pain, frustration, ambitions, expectations and accompanying physical imbalances. It is an in-depth look into the root cause of the author developing endometriosis.

If there is anything to know about endometriosis, it's that it is painful, physically painful. And so are many autoimmune disorders affecting 90% of women worldwide. They can be painful physically or mentally and this book is such an incredible read for anyone suffering from any form of pain and needing to go on living, pretending and hiding behind a cheerful face.

Despite dealing with pain, the author, Ania G., does not leave you feeling hopeless and desperate. Instead, this beautiful woman is determined to show you pain free living is possible and it requires your full engagement and commitment to letting go of the beliefs that don't serve you, adhering to a clean and healthy diet and regiments, reaching out for help and surrounding yourself with positive people.

Ania G has the ability to glamorize the disease and make you want to take action. She radiates with extremely motivating positivity and determination. Alone in the Crowd is a must read for anyone suffering from pain, especially endometriosis affecting so many women all over the world. It is a breeze of hope for them. If one woman can succeed, others can too.

Joanna Puciata

INHC, AADP, CGP, THCC,

*Author, Integrative Nutrition Health Coach, Certified Gluten Practitioner, Beauty Expert and Founder of Heal 'N Glow.*

# Words from the Author

I have always wanted to write a book that matters; a book that could make a change in people's lives, whether inspirational, motivational, or educational, or all in one.

I find endometriosis to be a huge mystery. It affects not just women, but our families, spouses, friends, and society at large. Yes, there are countless scientists and doctors working on finding the source of and cure for "endo" but as of this writing, there are only possibilities on the horizon. My dear friend, I am in your shoes; I live your life. I have a blog that you can read AniaLive.com where I blog about Endometriosis, living well, cooking, and nutrition. I have found medical approaches that can help; I have some great recipes and diet books. But until this book, I have never found anyone who would openly write about their own hardships connected to endometriosis. So I wrote to reach out to you and those around you. I wanted people to understand, without necessarily using professional medical terminology that the average person has never heard of.

I believe in passing things on. I have experienced things and learned things which I think are worth sharing. I believe my words can change your life. And it thrills me to know that I can make a difference for someone, somewhere.

Endometriosis is still a mystery and still so incredibly misunderstood, hence you cannot take the opinions of others as "gospel truth." You need to develop your own understanding and what works best for you, and I am here to help. You are and I am individuals, so there is no such thing as "one diagnosis fits all."

Life with endometriosis can be enjoyable, but this comes with much information, inspiration and huge determination. But if you are willing to do it, your life can be awesome! Knowledge, education, curiosity - these and more hold all the answers you need.

A portion of the proceeds from the sale of each book will go to support the ongoing efforts and work of [EndoPositive.org](EndoPositive.org) because I believe so strongly in what we are doing here. When you go to [AniaLive.com](AniaLive.com) you can easily purchase my book for yourself and a friend. When you go to AniaLive.com you can easily purchase my book for yourself and a friend.

Since English is not my first language you may hear my accent coming through in my writing. The best thing about this is, when we finally do meet, we'll feel like lifelong friends, right?

I am here for you, so feel free to contact me!    AniaLive.com

## I WAS A LITTLE GIRL IN PAIN

I lived in an unknown world of daily suffering. I didn't know why. I didn't know how I should express myself or how to be heard, understood and respected. I was optimistic, however, positive and happy on the outside as I didn't like being behind.

I was told I was lazy. That hurt. I had more x-rays than my grandma. I always knew something was wrong with me, but I did not know what. I was a child. It was not until 22 years later when my body finally gave up on me and my liver could not take any more pain killers, after a surgery and about to go for another I decided it was time for a change.

I took a close look at how we are treated and how little most experts know about endometriosis. Even the dictionary didn't know how to describe it. I didn't want doctors experimenting with me to TRY what might work for me or other women. I didn't feel it is ok for anyone to decide for me when and how often I should have surgery unless it was a life or death situation. I figured we know how to walk on the moon and create amazing tools and solve problems yet our understanding of endometriosis is far behind.

I read and researched everything to get my hands on to try and understand this nebulous disease and try to make sense of it for myself. I recruited doctors from every modality of health care. I took it all and made sense out of nonsense, what worked for me, and started living well with endometriosis. After I looked around and saw so many beautiful, hurt, troubled women all over the globe suffering physically and mentally because someone decided there was no cure for endometriosis. I decided to make a difference and prove otherwise. While others are still looking at how to perfect the surgeries I come and show you how to live well with no pain. I have launched a Worldwide Educational Organization: EndoPositive International™ Together, with Doctors from every medical discipline we educate not only patients but their families, mates and partners.

My goal is to make sure women are taken seriously – this is the most important matter to me. Armed with personal knowledge about endometriosis and our bodies we can all better prevent this disease from ravaging out bodies and our minds and we can stop believing we are crazy. Every woman will respond to this knowledge differently, but those who choose to accept ownership of their bodies and their lives can and will implement healthy changes and positive reinforcements that will help them to live well with endometriosis and become an advocate for living well to inspire other women.

To me awareness is truly making a difference, not only collecting signatures and giving a platform for voices. Together we will make a difference, I promise! Like no one else out there we can confidently say: I understand you as I was in your shoes. And I am not the only one who today can enjoy more of a pain free life.

Be confident, you can do it, and EndoPositive International™ is where you can learn how and where your voice can be heard. With lots of love, your Endo sister Ania G.

Founder of [EndoPositive International™](EndoPositive International) Empowering the 175 million women globally who suffer from Endometriosis, giving them a stage – giving them a voice.

# Prologue

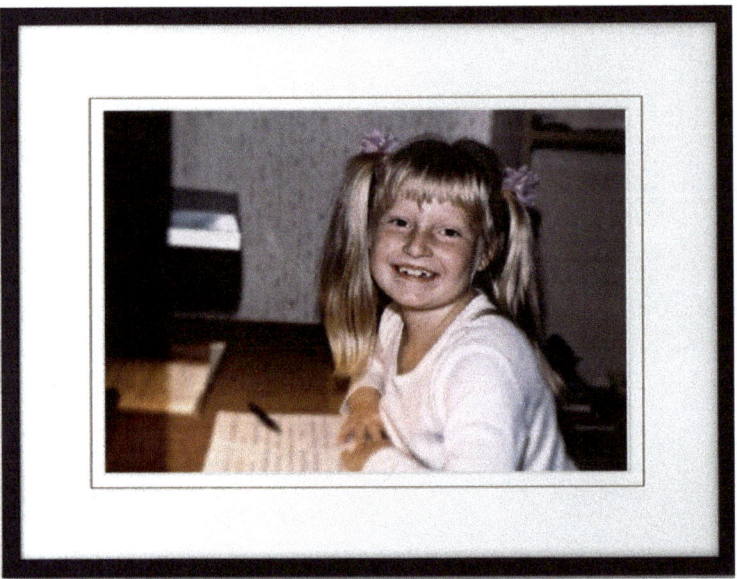

Everyone scrambled back to their seats as the door burst open. The director marched into the classroom and glanced around. I could see something in her eyes that I hadn't seen before—anger? Or fear? Finally, she cleared her throat. "Not a word from anyone… and stay in your seats. Nobody moves until I come back - understood?"
She glared at us one last time, then turned and left, pulling the classroom door shut behind her.

It was a beautiful spring day in April 1986. I was 8 years old. I had enjoyed the walk to school with my friend Adele. The first class was art, but when we got into the classroom, the teacher wasn't there. We didn't mind. It was common for a teacher to be a few minutes late, so we continued to play. The boys were running around making noise and throwing paper planes at each other and we, girls, were talking and laughing. Pretty soon we realized that our teacher was later than usual. In such cases, the class representative was supposed to go to the teacher office to see if we were going to get a sub, if we were to go home, or if we were just to continue waiting.

Just then the Director entered and told us to wait. This wasn't normal. Something was happening. But we didn't have any idea what it was.

As we waited, everyone started to get quiet. Pretty soon, the room was silent. As the minutes passed, I breathed out a deep breath, then let my mind drift outside to the playground—to the soft April breeze and sunshine, to the sounds of my playmates scampering around and calling to each other—before fear of the unknown, of my teacher missing, and the stillness in the room grabbed me by the neck and yanked me back to the present. Finally, one of the girls at the back of the room said in a hushed voice, "What do you think? What is going on?"

"Last time this happened we were told of a train that killed three of our classmates," one of the boys replied. We sat in silence as we thought about what might have happened. Soon, a murmur arose, as we tossed ideas back and forth—then the door opened and our mouths slammed shut. The director stood at the door, her hands on her hips. "What did I tell you...no talking! Listen, all of you, pack of your stuff, your books, and your personal belongings, and leave the school premises right away. Don't dawdle, don't push your friends or act up—and don't cause a panic. Stay together until you are close to your homes, then go straight inside. Do not stop anywhere or speak to anyone one."

We stared silently as she continued, "All of you look outside the window. You can see there was an accident at the railway. The air is very polluted, and we are out of masks, so cover your faces with your garments. Now move, all of you!"

She closed the door behind her and silence hung in the air for a few moments. Then, like good little soldiers, we gathered our things and marched, single file, out of the class and joined the other silent students marching down the hallway. The quietness in the classroom was so loud I could hear the clock that hung above the blackboard at the front of the room ticking.

Outside, the air seemed fine to me. The sun was still beaming its warmth and there was no odor. But I knew better than to question the director. School was very crowded and everyone was walking towards the door. We made it through crowded hallways and doors; we were out in the fresh spring air, yet we were covering our faces as needed. As kids do, we began taking deep breathes just for fun and to show everybody nothing would happen to us anyway.

"Ania, wait!" Piotrus, my older brother by five years, ran up behind me and grabbed my shoulder, loosening my gray sweater arms from around my mouth.

"Piotrus! You know what the director said!" I quickly tightened the sweater knot behind my head. He linked his arm in mine and we quickened our pace towards home, not saying another word.

"We'll have to wait for Mamma and Pappa to tell us what has happened. But I know there was a big explosion at the railway," Piotrus said, as he closed the front door of our "row home" behind me. We headed to our bedroom to put our belongings away. Momma kept the house neat and we did not dare leave anything out in the open.

We spent the rest of the afternoon playing in his room. Our television had only two channels, and watching the news was not something children did. There wasn't anything on until 7:15 that we wanted to see anyway. At that time, we would watch cartoons and then head to bed. So we just played games and talked, waiting for Momma and Pappa to come home from work at 5:30. But today, they arrived home at noon. They whispered to each other as Momma hung her coat up in the tiny closet, and nodded at my brother and me as we stood in the entrance to the living room. I knew better than to ask questions. Children in Poland were not allowed to ask questions, nor engage an adult in conversation, unless asked to do so.

"Make sure you get enough of 'it'," Momma said to Pappa as he left the house. She closed the door behind him and the fear on her face reached out and grabbed my stomach. I stifled a gasp. Even though I trusted my parents, I wanted, needed, to know what was happening. But Momma simply brushed passed us and headed to the kitchen. A short time later, I heard the front door open. A few seconds later, Pappa entered the kitchen, and placed a bottle on the faded wooden kitchen table. Both Momma and I turned to face him.

"Piotrus, come here," Momma called out. "Ania, sit at the table. Pappa, take your seat too." We all sat down, then Momma grabbed a spoon from the drawer beside the stove, walked over, picked up the bottle then set both in front of Pappa. "You go first." Mamma crossed her arms in front of her chest.

Pappa quickly took two spoonsful, his face scrunching up like he had just sucked on a lemon. Mamma nodded at my brother, who followed Pappa's lead. Then it was my turn.

I turned the bottle so that I could read the label. L-u-g-o-l. I had never heard of it before, but I didn't dare ask what it was. Instead, I obediently gulped my two spoonsful, the liquid burning down my throat into my stomach. I retched, but held it down. Mamma nodded at me; then she quickly choked back her dose of the red liquid.

I didn't know for a long time what was this liquid for and then I frankly didn't care; I trusted my parents. I think my parents were scared, and I am not sure they knew what there were doing. But it looked to me as if they had to make a fast decision. There was no time to think; they needed to act.

We drank the liquid and that was it. No explanation, no telling us what happened at the train station, nothing but, "Now go play in your rooms."

As I lay in bed that evening, I caught snippets of news from the television as the sound emanated through my open bedroom door. "Explosion at the plant station…radio activity…Chernobyl…."

It was impossible for me to know the impact these words would have on me as I grew up. That day changed my life entirely! Not just my life, but the lives of many people.

I never heard another word about that day in April. But eventually there would be another word that would be directly linked to that fateful day, a word that would throw my world into turmoil, causing me endless pain, heartache, and sleepless nights in my twenties and thirties.

## ENDOMETRIOSIS

The word "endometriosis" comes from the Latin word "endometrium", which is the tissue that lines the uterus. The menstrual cycle, this tissue builds up and is shed if she does not become pregnant.

But with endometriosis, the tissue develops outside the uterus, usually on other reproductive organs inside the pelvis or in the abdominal cavity.

Each month, this misplaced tissue responds to the hormonal changes of the menstrual cycle by building up and breaking down, just as the endometrium does, resulting in internal bleeding.

In endometriosis, displaced endometrial tissue continues to act as it normally would - it thickens, breaks down, and bleeds with each menstrual cycle. Because this displaced tissue has no way to exit a woman's body, it becomes trapped. Thus, unlike menstrual fluid from the uterus that is shed by the body, blood from the misplaced tissue surrounding the endometriosis becoming inflamed or swollen.

This process can cause irritation, eventually producing scar tissue around the area that may develop into lesions or growths - abnormal tissue that binds organs together.

In some cases, particularly when an ovary is involved, the blood can become embedded in the tissue where it is located, forming blood blisters the may become surrounded by a fibrous cyst.

Endometriosis most commonly involves the ovaries, bowel, or the tissue lining the pelvis. When the ovaries are affected, cysts called endometriomas may form. Endometrial tissue may spread beyond the pelvic region. It can affect all areas of the body, including the kidneys and the bladder, because cells are continuously growing outside the uterus.

# ALONE IN THE CROWD

## LIVING WELL WITH ENDOMETRIOSIS

# CHAPTER 1 | Coming to America

Before I get into how endometriosis changed my life, I want to share a little of my background. Being Polish, education was the biggest part of my childhood. While growing up in my homeland, we were not allowed to be children in the same way American children are. We rarely played outside, and we were allowed to have friends over only when our parents relented. You have to remember, when I grew up in Poland, it was communist. We had curfew at 7 pm. We weren't allowed outside after 7 pm or we could be shot by soldiers. School work and somber faces ruled our world, and I grew up shy, but with a mind of my own. At age 13, I had already decided I wanted to live in the United States. This decision came quickly after a family trip to Norway.

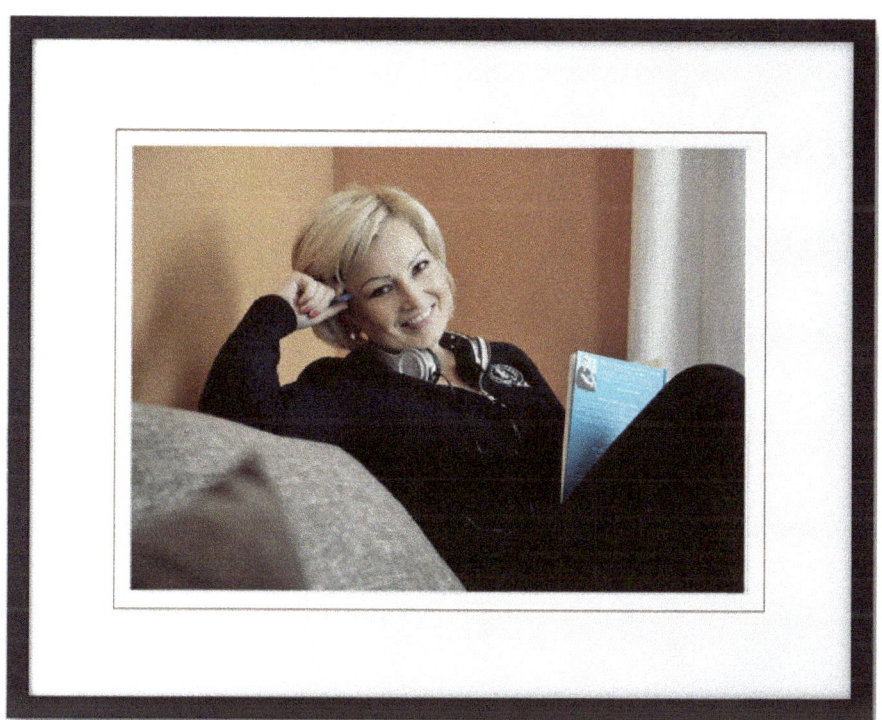

## A DIFFERENT WAY OF LIFE

While in Norway, I realized that people lived a different and better life. They were free. It was so noticeable, people actually had smiles on their faces. When I entered a store, I could not believe the diverse selections, including so many kinds of fruits and vegetables. Some were already actually pilled or cut in pieces ready for eating. And the variety of chocolates and candies just blew my mind! I instantly recalled my notebook full of colorful candy wrappers. It was a game all my girlfriends played. We collected chocolate and candy wraps because candy was a rare treat. (The boys collected soda and beer cans.)

I could not believe such a variety of food existed! But my heart quickly sank knowing that back home, the stores offered limited amenities such as bread, vinegar, and milk. The only time we had specialties such as bananas and oranges was around Christmas time. When we shopped, we stood in long lines, hoping that something might be left when our turn came to enter the store.

I can remember on one occasion when my mother wanted to buy Piotrus a bike. She waited in line for over five hours. If we wanted to buy a refrigerator or a washing machine, the line would be so long that we had to hire people to stand in line for us.

The trip to Norway fueled my determination to leave Poland. I wanted a better life. I wanted to experience something new and something exciting. For the first time, I felt that life was limitless!

## ON TO AMERICA

Fortunately, my parents were visionaries and they deposited a strong foundation for their children to build upon. Thus, at 22 after graduating from the University of Pedagogics (Education) and Psychology in Bialystok with a Bachelor's Degree in Fashion and Design and Master's Degree in Psychology and Education, I applied for and was granted an immigration visa to America.

## FREEDOM AND INDEPENDENCE

I could taste these in the air the moment I disembarked Lufthansa at New York's LaGuardia International Airport. I then rented a car and headed for Maryland, where I stayed with a friend, Yoni. She was the manager of the beachwear store where I eventually worked. (I first worked in a restaurant.)

Three months after my arrival, Yoni and I took a trip to Marco Island, Florida. It was love at first sight; I had found my paradise! The culture, the language, the lush homes, and unique and beautiful botany intoxicated me, and soon we settled in a rented condo on the island. We even had a community swimming pool, and I called everyone I knew back in Poland to let them know how happy I was.

Quickly assimilating into the culture, I reveled in the European flavor. People dressed in trendy fashions, and everywhere I turned someone offered me a handshake, a smile, or an encouraging word. I soon found a job at a retail store selling clothing, where I could also develop my English.

It is true that one person's heart truly "knows" another, and people recognized my abilities and talent almost immediately I was fortunate to meet people who were generous, kind, and patient. I became an excellent sales person, engaging into conversation during business transactions; I felt as if my job was entertainment.

When my boss recognized my people skills, I was given a higher position only a couple weeks after being hired. My ability to win over difficult customers and handle touchy situations deepened my boss's trust in me. When he promoted me to manager, I felt like I was running my own business. I felt like I had it all - almost.

The one thing I missed was my family: dad, mom, my grandparents, and my brother and sisters. I longed for them to join me and experience what real life was like. As the weeks and months passed, I yearned to have them with me, and I made it my mission to bring them over as soon as possible.

## RECOGNIZING MY GIFTS

I have always gravitated towards people who are older and more mature, and my friends in Marco Island were no different. For instance, my friend, Yoni, is a sweet lady, around my mom's age. Even though she's returned to her homeland of Israel, we are still in touch and I am friends with her children.

Yoni was the first person to tell me there was something different, something special about me. I had never thought of myself in this way before; in Poland, we were taught to confirm, to be a face in the crowd. Although my parents were great encouragers, I had believed the ruling party line: follow the rules; conform to what is expected; become a faceless face in the crowd. Yoni, however, saw deep within me. "You're going to make a difference in this world," she would tell me. "You're going to be someone special."

I would giggle at her words, not knowing how to reply.

While working with Yoni in the beachwear store, I started looking for another job; not because I didn't like what I was doing, but I was ready to try something new, to raise my bar higher. One day, while walking by a shopping plaza on Marco Island, I saw a beautiful evening dress that caught my attention. I decided to walk into a store and check it out. I opened the door and - wow! I was amazed at the beautiful array of clothing. I fell in love with the amazing attire, and felt like I was in a movie. All that was needed to make my day dreaming complete was a piano and some smooth jazz music.

A sales person approached me and we started talking. "Where are you from?" she soon asked.

I hung my head, as if something was wrong. "Poland."

When I glanced up at the sales lady, she smiled. "The owner is a Russian woman, and I'm sure she would like to meet you."

I met Tanya, the store owner and a beautiful woman, soon after that. We quickly struck up a friendship, and she immediately hired me. (We are still friends today, and I'm thankful she is such a big part of my life.) Coming to work every day made me feel like a princess with the best clothing available at my fingertips.

## SHARING WITH FAMILY

After three years, I saved enough money to bring my family to live with me. I had rented a four-bedroom home with a large patio and a pool. My sister, Jo, came first. She was 18 and five years younger than me, so I took over being her mother, and had to learn very quickly how to deal with teenagers. But as I look back, Jo and I had some great times, with lots of tears and laughter.

When my dad, mom, and grandparents joined us a few months later, countless tears of joy were spilled and endless hugs were shared. My parents– Mom, Ala, a dentist by profession; Dad, Jurek or George, an economist; Asia, my younger sister by five years; my older brother

Piotrus or Peter, and my grandparents, Frank and Henia—were soon buckled up in the van I had rented. As we left LaGuardia Airport and headed to Florida, memories of my first days in this wonderful country flashed through my mind. Truly I was in the "home of the free."

After we settled in at my home, our lives seemed "larger than life." Watching my family experience such an exotic lifestyle—oranges, coconuts, and alligators amazed them—thrilled my heart. And the first time my grandmother opened the fridge and saw the variety of food, I thought she was going to keel over from shock!

While I worked, they explored the island and all it had to offer. However, they did not understand that land was privately owned, and they marveled that I owned the house we all lived in.

"And the stores too, they are owned by someone?" asked my grandfather. His words made me realize just how fortunate I was to live in this great land.

At times it was scary to leave my family unattended, as I never knew what ideas might pop into their heads. For instance, my grandfather asked me to buy him a fishing rod, and I thought he wanted to fish in the canal in front of our house. I soon found out he was going to our neighbors! Grandfather didn't speak English, so I do not know how he made this deal, but the neighbors allowed him to come over anytime he wanted.

Asia and Peter quickly settled in; Asia found a job in a retail store and Peter started his own enterprise. With everyone working, Mom and Dad returned to Poland, but they still come for periodic vacations. Realizing how much they all enjoyed living here fueled my determination to work hard so they could enjoy their new lives. It was my time to give it back to them. Although I had been raised in a solemn and dour society, my parents and grandparents had done their best to provide a happy childhood.

All too soon another year had passed, and, sadly I had to make the decision to return to Poland to finish my degree. But I now knew what freedom looked and tasted like; and I would be back as soon as I could to this new country I loved so much.

## MY FAMILY HISTORY

I grew up in a modest home in Poland, similar to a two-bedroom apartment in America. It was an average but adequate house. We lived in the city of Bialystok and owned a compact car, a Squere. Similar to much of Europe, most of what we needed was within walking distance, so the car was rarely used. Cows and horses were common in the market or the local square. While shopping in the streets, you could find fresh eggs and milk in a can, straight from the farm.

My father came from the village Plociczno near a beautiful town called Elk. The region is still called "lungs of Poland" because of its many lakes and forests. We had a summer home, in Elk, and my siblings and I spent childhood summers there. My grandfather was a bee keeper and a farmer, and also raised chickens, goats, and cows. My Grandfather's book coming out in 2015 www. We learned much working on the farm, but the greatest experience was gaining wisdom from those who were older.

My parents taught us how to act and how to communicate with our elders. When guests arrived at our home, my parents always encouraged us to join them, something I could not tell my friends for fear of reprisal. It was an opportunity to listen and learn from mature people, ones who had accomplished things in their lives.

Being around my grandparents in the village was a time to expand and develop. We engaged in intellectual conversations, discovering principles necessary for our future. We were encouraged to read books. Grandfather would read us stories from the Bible and teach us valuable life lessons. We would also visit friends of my grandparents and sit and observe, something my grandfather diligently instilled in us.

My grandfather also took me fishing. It was not a typical boat; it was more like pieces of wood meshed to serve as a floating device. By 5 am, we would be out on the lake, casting our net and hauling up fish. As a 12-year-old, I learned to paddle a small craft in the wind and the rain.

My father was much the same as my grandfather. Each day presented opportunities for lessons about life. If he worked on the family car, he would take me with him and explain the various parts of an engine, while showing me how to fix it. I though he was crazy! What young girl wants to learn about cars? However, today, when a mechanic tells me about a transmission, I know what he is talking about, and no one can take advantage of me.

My mom did the same. She would take me to work at her dentist's office. Whether making dentures or examining someone's teeth, she would teach me the numbers pertaining to each tooth and their function. I watched my mother cook for parties and family events, learning her techniques and methods. These lessons came in handy whenever I spent time with my grandfather and grandmother.

My childhood was not one that most American children would understand. I only had one doll, not because I was deprived but because that was how it was in Poland. Instead, I learned how to be creative and use my imagination. I also spent more time learning and developing myself for adulthood, rather than having fun. Despite my parents' best efforts to give me a pleasant upbringing, I still lived in a country that was gray - the people, the weather, the landscape, and even any sense of hope. By gray, I refer to the mood of the country and the limited opportunities.

In Poland, expectation was a word you rarely heard. The future was not something you dreamed about; it was something you accepted. It might be surprising, but people who have lived in that type of atmosphere actually enjoyed it, believing it was the right way to live. If anyone heard that you, as an individual, were happy and smiling, these people would shake their heads, as if something was wrong with you. Sadly, there were thousands of Eastern Block people immigrating to Poland because they thought we had "paradise" in our hands.

At age 13, I had already decided I wanted to live like the people I had seen in Norway. I no longer wanted a doll that was gray with a gray dress or a pencil that was gray. I wanted a doll with rosy cheeks, a pink dress, and even a pink pencil!

That same summer, I realized I could be different was a life-changing time for me. At school, we were required to wear a navy blue uniform. Everyone was the same, no exceptions. But I was going to be the exception! I wanted to explore my potential. There was only one way I could do that: I had to leave the country. I also knew that those who did leave never returned.

It was not only Norway that held such promise to me; all of Western Europe held out the promise of hope. Traveling from Belgium to Germany, it was easy to see how vastly superior their lifestyles were. Those outside my family who knew my desire to leave the country blamed it on the fact I that I did not like the cold. There was even a time that I agreed that the weather determined my feelings.

As I advanced into my teen years, I realized that Poland was a beautiful country, with a great culture, gorgeous scenery, great food, and hospitable people. When someone enters a Polish home, they are made to feel like honored guests, with the best that home had to offer at their disposal.

Weddings began at 7 pm and often did not end until 5 am. Many of the guests would not have any shoes on because they had been dancing all night.

But my feelings towards my country went beyond the nicely wrapped package that visitors saw. In everyday life, people seemed to live to complain. If an average person was asked how they were doing, the other person had best have at least two hours to hear all the complaints. Complaints about sickness, about the weather, about the neighbor's dog, the runaway horse, the hole in the roof...they went on and on. If someone ever said they were doing "fine," that person would be complained about to a neighbor or a family member. To say you were doing "fine" drew the ire and jealousy of others. And to even mention the thought of starting a new enterprise met with every reason imaginable as to why the endeavor would never work.

As I entered my late teens, the continual negativity that pervaded the culture drove my determination to leave even deeper within me. My if-something-is-not- working-then-do-something-to-change-or-fix-it attitude made me an island in my own country.

This may sound really crazy, but my father used to tell me, "You know there is only one thing you cannot do; open an umbrella in your butt." As funny as that sounds, I took that seriously. I never took "no" for an answer. If somebody and told me, "You can't do that!" I was even more determined to do it. Nothing is impossible was and still is my motto. I believe that if you have a problem of any nature, you need to attempt to solve it. It's okay to fail; if you try and you fail you can always try again and find a way to do it better. Problems are meant to be faced head on, no backing down, with the resiliency to find a way to succeed.

Albert Einstein said, "Never give up on what you really want to do. The person with big dreams is more powerful than one with all the facts." I was a dreamer, a powerful person, and I was going to fulfill my dreams.

## LEARNING TO QUESTION

While living in Poland, there was a stigma that was part of the culture: If you asked a question, you were considered a dumb person. Questions were not allowed; you had to know everything or at least pretend to. In school, we were lectured for an hour each class. When the teacher had finished speaking he/she would ask, "Do you have any questions?" No one dared raise a hand. Even if a student had their own idea about a subject or a different point of view, or felt like challenging the teacher's presentation, it was better to remain silent. What if the question confused or embarrassed the teacher because he/she did not know how to answer? Such questions would label the student as a rebel, a non-conformist, and would be subject to reprisals.

I carried this stigma with me during my first weeks in America. But I quickly learned that it was okay to question, to wonder, to offer personal opinions and viewpoints. I felt like someone had popped the cork of a champagne bottle; my questions soon came bubbling out to anyone and everyone. I was coming to life. I was free to explore, to dream, to live life as I was meant to live it, with no limitations. In America, questions showed interest; they gained insight and understanding. Even today, I like to delve into conversations in which questions are asked and answered, and knowledge is freely shared. To me, this is the essence of life.

Questions allow people to open a door to their lives. "Do you mind if…?" "What do you think of…?" "What about…" "Have you ever thought of…?" As I became acclimatized to American culture, I found people were always willing to answer my questions, to engage in conversations in which we both learned and grew. Such conversations are food for the mind; they are wealth for the soul; they stimulate the spirit, bring the entire person alive.

While working at the beachwear store, then at the dress store, I would smile at my customers and ask, "How are you doing today?" Rarely did I start out by asking what clothing might interest them. I wanted to know who they were as a person first. Doing so naturally led to a particular piece of clothing or an accessory. At the cash register, both the customer and I felt good about our time together.

Asking questions led me to an epiphany: I discovered nothing was impossible. It was amazing. If I was shopping at a store, eating at a restaurant, or out for a night with friends, I would ask a question and people seemed to want to rush to answer, or to offer me assistance. I think sometimes when people looked at me, I looked as if wanted to ask question! Sometimes, even before I opened my mouth, someone was already by my side, offering answers, advice, or directions. I no longer felt like I was dumb. People fascinated me, and I, in turn, seemed to fascinate them.

## CONQUERING MY FEARS

But all of that came with time. I had earned by degree in my home university, and two friends, Agnieszka and Ula, and my sister had moved back to America with me. As I mentioned, when I came to America, my first job was working at a restaurant. I quickly discovered the people spoke fast, too fast, and with different accents, for me to fully comprehend what was being said. Fear gripped my heart because I did not know the language well, and life moved at such a fast pace. I felt overwhelmed and unsure. But within a few days, my determination to succeed soon dominated my fears. . However, I still feared asking questions. Even though I had learned to speak English back home, it was quite different in America.

My friends spoke only a few words and phrases of English, such as yes, no, thank you, please and I can do that.

"Let's try to find work at this restaurant," I said, pointing one across the street. They both agreed.

"My friends and I are looking for work; do you have anything?" I asked the man who greeted us at the restaurant. He stared at me, then my friends, for a few moments. I froze. Did I say something wrong? Then he nodded and handed me a stack of papers. He then talked so fast, I barely understood what he wanted us to do. "Come back tomorrow." "Okay, okay no problem." I replied, smiling. However, as we left the restaurant and headed back to my apartment, I thought to myself, Oh my God, what am I gonna do now?

The four of us went home, and using a dictionary, we looked up every word in our job applications. It literally took us all night. We went back the next day, and were immediately employed in the kitchen. But we almost didn't make it through our first shift.

The other workers, trying to be helping, gave us directions. "Do this. Go there. This belongs over there. No, we do it this way." I felt like I was trapped on a freeway of words and couldn't keep up. After an hour, my friends and I were exhausted. We did not have time to waste learning, but we didn't have a choice but to go slow. In some ways, I was like a parrot repeating words I heard without truly knowing the meaning or the context of what was being said.

We worked with several African Americans, something that was a new experience; there were only a handful of colored people living in Poland during my years there. As helpful as they tried to be, I had difficulty with their accent. Then I made an almost fatal mistake.

An African American in Poland was referred to as a "nigger," and I did not realize how offensive this word was. I was cutting vegetables side by side with an African American, and halfway through our attempt at conversing he said, "Why are you being so nice to me?"

"Because we have no niggers in Poland," I replied, and tossed some carrots into a pot.

"What did you call me?" he said, his eyes ablaze with anger.
"A nigger," I replied and shrugged.

He waved his knife in front of my nose. "I am not a nigger, I am a black man." He never spoke to me after that.

The next day, I brought my Polish dictionary to work and showed him the definition, and apologized for offending him. I just did not know that the word was offensive.

## LEARNING EXPERIENCES

I wanted to make friends, so I talked as much as possible. Most people thought my accent was funny. They embraced me as someone from a new culture, but there were funny moments. For instance, someone asked me if I liked "grass." I innocently responded by saying, "Yes, green grass is very pretty." Before that day, no one ever asked me if I liked grass, and frankly, I did not find anything particular about it. Then I found that grass was marijuana. I was learning words, good and bad.

My innocence must have seemed peculiar to many people as well. I had never cussed before; I would never have thought of stealing, cheating, or lying. I was brought up to respect people, to be kind, to be fair, and have integrity. I thought everyone was that way. Fortunately, no one tried to take advantage of my good nature.

## FINDING MYSELF

After a few months of working as a waitress, a man came in and told me I was too good to work there. He wanted to hire me for his business.

"What do you do?" I asked.

He said he had a beachwear retail store, and wanted me to work as a salesperson.

"How would you know I would be good candidate for this job? You do not know me."

"I like the way you present yourself," he replied and hired me on the spot. This job opened many doors for me. I met many people from all over the world, and I learned that if I wanted to do anything in America, if I worked hard and believed, I could make my dreams come true.

These people believed in me as I believed in myself. I began to open up and was willing to learn what they had to teach me. My English improved over time, and I loved working with customers. I learned that it was not about selling a product; I was to sell myself.

## WALKING THROUGH OPEN DOORS

One day, while working in the retail store, a black man entered the store and he walked up to me.

"I would like to hire you," he said.

"What do you do?"

"I am a potential candidate for the President of."….. he went on to name a large African Nation.

"What would you like me to do? I'm just a salesperson."

He said that he wanted me to help run his presidential campaign here in the United States. However, I objected and explained that I did not know anyone. Nevertheless, he insisted on hiring me. I agreed to give think about it and told him I would call him back. When he walked away, I thought to myself, He must be joking. I did not take him seriously because I was learning that not everyone who tells me something actually means it.

Two weeks later, we spoke on the phone and he convinced me to work for him, and, as his confidence in me grew, he gave me greater responsibility, working with well-known public figures. (Due to confidentially, I cannot name these people.) Over time, I began to meet important people such as diplomats and officials in government. What an interesting twist of fate; this was probably the most unusual job I've ever had in my twelve years of living in America.

While working for this man and his Presidential campaign, I learned never to give up, to keep an open mind, and not to immediately reject a proposal from anyone. I learned that I can discover things from anyone, no matter their importance. Yes, there is positive and negative teaching, but I loved people and loved talking to them, learning more about them and their culture. Most of all, I loved helping people.

It is so important to have compassion and a willingness to help. It's important to learn and to share with others. To go through good times and bad, and learn all you can from the experience.

I believe that no matter where you are born, whether you are sick or healthy, rich or poor, you can find your way through any circumstance if you set your mind and heart to do so. Life is up to each individual; we all have free will and choice. We all have the power to make life-changing decisions, whether for good or bad. No one can take the power of choice away; it is part of who we are as human beings.

I believe there are countless people in the world like me, people who are looking for answers and encouragement, people who are hungry for knowledge and life's experiences. We can learn from each other, grow from each other's lessons. We can change for the good and make life better for everyone we come in contact with.

## WE CAN DO ANYTHING

The story of how I learned to speak English has a lot to do with my belief that we can do anything we set our minds to do. My grandmother had an elderly woman friend, Dagny, who used to be a well-known actress. One time, my grandmother took me to visit her, and I found out that she was teaching English. I got so excited when I heard her say that! She asked me if I would like to learn English, and without thinking of what it would cost, I answered immediately, "Yes!"

At ten-years-old, I did not think I needed anyone's permission. I knew that, somehow, I would figure it out with my parents. When I think about it today, that was a brave decision.

Actually, I really did not care how much it would cost my parents. I just wanted to learn English. My grandmother made an appointment for me to return the following week. I cannot explain the extreme connection I felt with her. I knew she was changing my life. After my fifth lesson, Dagny called my grandmother and said, "This girl is amazing. She has great talent." One day she looked me straight in the eyes and said, "God gave you talent; do not waste it." I was raised to respect God and I did not dare to disappoint Him. I took that very seriously.

Before I started learning English, I was very shy. Learning English was the first time I believed in myself. I finally believed that I was someone special and could do something special. Dagny made me feel very special. I talked to her about what I felt and what I thought. She listened, unlike all the teachers at school. Dagny made me believe, made me strong, and made me realize that following my dreams was the right path to take in life.

My English teacher and mentor had a huge impact on my life. Dagny taught me how to approach people. She taught me how to be motivated. She taught me how to influence people by loving them. I learned never to discard anybody. I wanted to inspire people to believe in themselves, and they could be whatever they wanted to be. I also told each student, "It does not matter what you do as long as you do it with love."

Dagny was amazed that I could learn English so fast. After two months, she said she had never had a student who had made such progress. I started taking English classes when I was 13, and after two years of classes I was teaching other Polish children. By age 15, I was fluent and teaching English with great success.

I must explain something: My English was not the same as American English, but followed British pronunciations, spelling, and grammar. While I wasn't fluent enough to speak easily as soon as I came to America, I had a greater understanding of English than most Polish people, so I could teach others. As my confidence grew, I realized I had another love – the love of passing knowledge onto others.

The students to whom I taught English became the best in their classes at school. They came to me twice a week for tutoring. I was not trying to make money, but I was paid for teaching the classes. For me, it was more than teaching English classes. This was another powerful lesson I learned early in life: do what you are passionate about and money will come to you. I was teaching these students to believe in themselves. I did exactly what Dagny did to me – I motivated and inspired.

One of my students, Anna, was super shy, small, and tiny. She had a very difficult time, and was one of the worst students in her class. Yet, she had an amazing talent. As a ballerina, she loved to dance and could do so like a feather. However, she hated English. Yet after a couple weeks in classes, her mom called and said to me, "I have never seen my daughter so happy." Anna loved coming to my class just so she could be with me.

The fact that Anna did not like English in the beginning did not matter to me. I wanted to help her because she had such a great attitude. If I told her to write an English word 100 times, she would do it. She was amazing. For instance, she would have to write the word "apple" many times because she would forget that there are two "p's" in it. Nevertheless, she would write it repeatedly and was always happy to do so. This brought me great joy.

## PEOPLE COME FIRST

When Dagny finally passed away, I felt like a part of me died. To honor her memory, I knew I needed to pass on what she had taught me. I needed to teach others to create change in their lives and move into action. I learned that life was really all about people. Not about things. Not about places. People are most important. Connecting emotionally with people creates relationships, and relationships make life worth living.

Most people are lacking love. People think they must have possessions to be happy such as money, property, and position. But no matter how much one accumulates, or what position one reaches, without love, without relationships, without family and friends, life is empty. These are the lessons I brought with me to America, lessons that have kept me strong, kept my heart pure, and help me to see the good in everyone I meet.

# CHAPTER 2 | *Facing the Enemy*

It might seem like my life has been filled with success. It has, but it has also had its share of pain and sadness. Part of that pain is the result of that fateful day in April 1986 when the Director sent all of us home from school.
But before I go into that, I have learned that no matter what happens in life, you need to live it to the fullest with no regrets. My life is all about caring, sharing, and helping others. For some reason, I always attract people who have issues and problems, insecurities. Nevertheless, they are not a burden to me, but a blessing.

It is most important to never disregard or judge someone for any reason. And the same goes for trials, for struggles, for the hard times we face in life. I've learned that "people are never the problem: viewpoints and attitudes are."

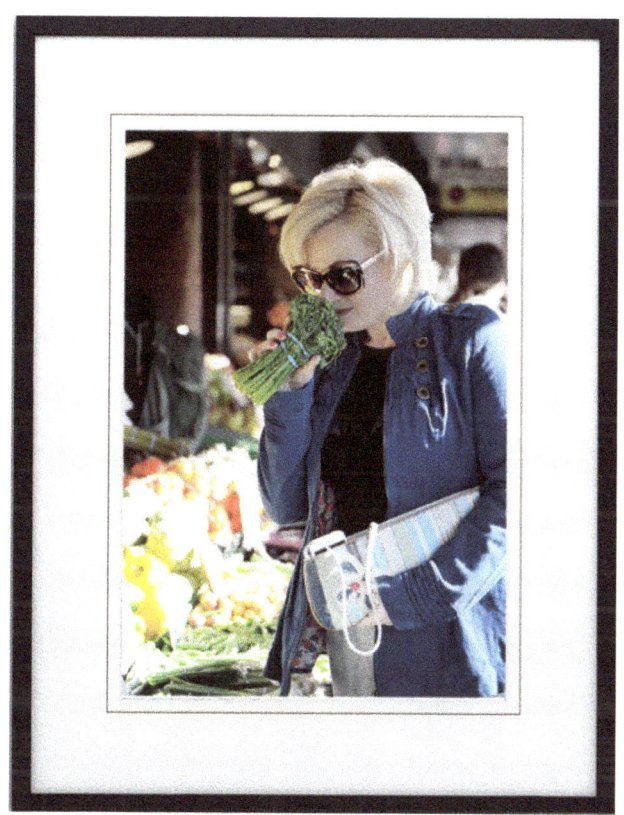

For example, when I come across someone who is moody or negative, I realize this person is struggling within themselves; something bad has or is happening to them. I've learned to look past what I see on the outside and to help that person see what is in their hearts. What is causing them to feel so down? So angry? So negative? Taking time to help someone gain a new perspective, offer help, or even something as simple as, "You're going to make it through" makes me feel alive, because I've contributed to someone's wellbeing.

### SHOOTING FOR THE STARS

I fly through my life like a rocket. I speed like crazy and I shoot for the stars. Sometimes, I hit the wall; it happens. Sometimes I fall but then, I get up again ready to shine like the sun peeking over the horizon for a new day. Obstacles and roadblocks present a choice - do I go over or around them? I choose to use them as stepping-stones to where I am headed. I see much of life as a choice; I get to choose my attitude, my direction, my purpose.

Pauses in life—those places where you cannot move forward, but must wait for something to change—are times to recoup, to reflect, to ponder, to change, to rest, refresh and recharge. Taking a break in life should be your choice to do so, not because you allowed what is in front of you to prevent you from moving forward. Just like daylight gives way to night time, pauses in life are chances to close your eyes and rest.

I also believe that our upbringing, our culture, shape us; we are a byproduct of our parents, our extended family, even our friends. We represent different behaviors and characteristics, which were modeled for us. Unfortunately, as much as we may be determined and ambitious, we cannot go against the natural laws of the universe, and sometimes we have to face things we never expected to face when we were just children. We wonder why things may go wrong, when we are doing what is right, what is good, what is helpful. We don't anticipate obstacles, especially when we are young and not familiar with the cycles of life. That was how it was with me.

I know that many of you have found this book because, like me, you have suffered from endometriosis. You are probably looking for some answers, solutions, and remedies. I know you may sit in your home dealing with it on your own, or trying to connect with others Online, not being able to connect with anyone who would relate to you. I know people think you are lazy or always grumpy. You are probably very often tired. You may have visited several doctors, researched many studies just to find anyone or anything you would identify yourself with.

## YOU ARE NOT ALONE

You are not alone. There are answers out there. You may start feeling better sooner that you imagine. I won't say there is one simple solution or one size fits all, as each case of our condition is very individual, but I believe together we can find answers and live fulfilled and joyful lives.

Let's Connect on Social Media. I want to connect with you on Social Media. If you reach out to me I will follow you back:

Twitter.com/AniaWrites
Instagram.com/AniaWrites
Linkedin.com/EndometriosisAuthorAniaG
Facebook.com/AuthorAniaG
Pinterest.com/AuthorAniaG
AniaLive.com

Also, remember you can connect with our growing movement of women around the world at EndoPositive.org. Here you can share your story and make an impact on other women who can benefit by hearing your story.

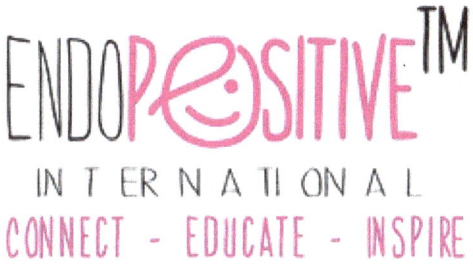

The more we share, the more powerful we become. The louder we speak, the more people will hear, the more we ask the more answers we will collect. The more we share, the bigger community we create. The bigger community we belong to, the less lonely we will be. The more doors we knock on, the more doors we will open.

I have looked for a long time for answers, for solutions, for people who would understand me, for doctors who could help me. That was a very long journey, completely on my own, completely strange, very difficult, extremely painful, sickening, and exhausting. But I have never given up. I have never stopped being curious. I have never stopped digging. I knew at some point getting through the stone age of unknown I would find a treasure of knowledge. I never allowed my misery to rob me of my precious life.

That's why I want to share the story of my life with you. I now know it began that fateful day in April when I was 8 years old. I am now 36 and have some answers that I hope will help you.

So let's begin this journey together!

## DREAMS AND GOALS

In my mid-twenties and living in Poland, I was living in town of Bialystok and was studying Psychology and Pedagogics at The University of Pedagogics (Education). I was also teaching English at that time. I had a clear view of who I wanted to be and where I was heading. Life was truly good. As an honors student, I had been given a scholarship to study in Nuremburg, Germany, for the Socrates Erasmus Program. What an honor - only eight students in my entire university of over 4,000 students were chosen for this program. Life was full of unlimited possibilities and I wanted to fulfill them all. I didn't plan on obstacles; in fact, I refused to see any. I would finish my degree, graduate, leave for the USA, and move to my next phase of life.

In the middle of my second university year, I was suddenly faced with something I had never dreamed would happen—limitations. I became tired and lethargic. I had to force myself to focus on my studies and put in extra effort to read and comprehend. Things took more time that they should and I grew increasing irritated. The thought about possibly staying behind and not being the top student was not going to be an option. I couldn't even think of not being able to perform. I didn't blame my setback on the way I felt; I blamed myself! Even though I couldn't define what was happening, nor did I suspect I was getting sick, I lived in denial of anything that might change my goals for me life. I just kept going - regardless. Even after graduating and moving to the USA, I continued to hide behind a façade of smiles and laughter when with others, while facing agonizing pain when alone.

## MY NEW "COMPANION"

From the very first days of living in Maryland, a new "companion" greeted me every morning - pain. It "greeted" me the moment I woke up; it stayed with me all day long; and it was the last thing I connected with before I feel asleep at night. I was exhausted, unsure, and had no idea what was happening to me. But I tried not to let the pain I felt in my body affect my mood and my interactions with people. I wanted to maintain my smile, my positive outlook. But bodily pain has a mind of its own. As days and weeks went by, it took its toll on my mental wellbeing. I felt something pressing against me, against my will, against my dreams and against my life. I had a new enemy, one I could not identify, and it was something within myself. My intention to live life to the fullest began to spiral downward. It was like owning a house that is suddenly destroyed by a hurricane.

I had no clue what was wrong. I only knew that distracting, damaging, disrupting pain was consuming my body. I felt it everywhere. It was all I could feel and talk about. I could not think, eat, sleep, or stay awake. I could not concentrate. I could not come up with answers because I didn't even have a clue where exactly the pain emanated from. For the first time since I was a little girl, I did not know how to deal with life. This was becoming my life's pattern. On the outside, things looked great, but on the inside, I was suffering. Days, months and years passed by, yet the pain didn't lessen, didn't go away. I was clueless, but could not, did not, dared not share what I was going through with anyone.

I struggled through the day at work, with only the thought of my bed awaiting me that kept me going. Once at home, I was bedridden. I could no longer do "life" anymore. What I have always despised was happening to me: I was trapped boxed in, limited, and restrained. I felt like a prisoner in chains, weighed down with burdens, and beyond exhaustion.

All I could see in the future was pain and hopelessness. I used to wake up in the morning with a good attitude. With a cup of coffee, I was ready for a new day. However, now, by the time I was done with my coffee, I was ready to go back to bed and sleep, hoping for some kind of relief. My smile was gone. My positive attitude abandoned me. My love for helping others disappeared. I was so weak, in so much pain, that I did not have the strength to pick up the telephone, call a friend, and tell them how much I was suffering. Finally, confused, helpless, and hurting, I finally realized I could not deal with this on my own.

## SOMETHING IS WRONG!!

At age 27, I had been in America for two years. But going to the doctor in a fairly new country was quite an experience. You are not sure you will understand all the terms, and you are not sure you will be understood. But I had to do something so I made an appointment. I had many tests run, and when I went back for the results, the doctor said, "All tests were perfectly fine. Would you like some pain killers? They will definitely help."

## I WAS FURIOUS!

I continued to read medical information and periodicals, trying to understand what was happening to me. With no insights, I was beginning to think I was going insane.

I tried several other doctors with the same results - no one could find the cause of my suffering. It was insulting, maddening, to hear the same answer over and over again. All the tests were negative; none showed any sign of an organ not working properly, or a virus or disease in my body. But the pain never subsided.

Most nights, I lay in my bed, curled up in a fetal position. I did not know what to do or where to go. I was heartbroken. I not only needed to uncover the cause of my pain, but I had to learn how to talk about it with my friends. This was the hardest part for me. I was always the one who was cheery and content. In fact, my nickname was "Sunshine." But now I was the one confused, searching for answers.

## AT THE BEGINNING

Looking back over my life, the pain in my body really began when I was a young girl. As I think back, I realize it began at age 13 after starting my menstruation. I actually think it has its beginning in that day in April 1986 when, as a young girl, I was exposed to radiation from the Chernobyl disaster, but I didn't know anything was wrong until a few years later.

I mention this because as a teenager, I tried to express my feelings, but was told I was too young to be tired, too young to have migraines or even headaches. Naturally I had to accept what others said: I was a good patriot of the "system." I remember complaining about headaches, but adults would laugh at me saying, "You don't even know what a headache is." Such is the Communist approach to human nature. You are told how to feel, what to think, how to act. Others know your body, your pain, better than you do. I have shivers thinking about this. It was like being in an army, following orders in regards to absolutely everything.

## DAILY PAIN

After moving to Marco Beach, my migraines became an almost daily affair. They served to deepen my pain, pain that crept through every inch of my body. I ached in my bones, in my skin, even the hair on my scalp hurt. I could not even file my fingernails because they hurt too. Covering my body with a blanket caused me to be in pain. Even wearing clothes caused my skin to be in horrible pain.

I was simply miserable. This was so depressing and disturbing.

As time went on, I found it difficult to walk. Nevertheless, I refused to give in or give up. I continued to work despite the agony I suffered. In order to be successful I had to keep my smile, my façade of self-confidence, and to dress to the "nines." I did my best not to show what I was going through. However, over time, my makeup would not cover the gray tones and shades. My image was changing; I was losing my beauty and vitality. I was changing right before my eyes, and I hated it.

Sometimes, I had to face comments such as, "Something is wrong with your face and eyes." "Are you drinking too much?" "Why are you staying out and partying all night?" None of these were true.
But something was definitely wrong.

## FIGHTING THE ENEMY

Every battle has an enemy. You must fight to win or you will lose. And I hated to lose. I had to fight every day to stay alive and be vibrant. But it was time to do my research, to start digging and finding answers. I would search and find a way out. Yet the more I looked, the more I found that no one could give me any direction or guidance. Frustration set in. Helplessness knocked on the door of my heart…but I was not going to give in.

When I first started to confide to others what I was going through, those closest to me thought I was sick because I was working too much. It was true I worked long hours. Due to my nature of taking on other people's burdens and problems, some suggested that I was simply overwhelmed. But I had never carried someone's problems. I did not believe in carrying extra baggage. Well-meaning people asked me to stop offering assistance or aid to others. However, I could not stop because this was like asking me to stop living. It was therapeutic to see other people getting better due to working with me. Remember I am a Psychologist by nature and by training. It is my nature to nurture others, patients and friends. To some extent, this was my way of dealing with my agonizing pain.

For me, the source of pain was my enemy, an unknown enemy. There is a saying: "Keep your friends close, but keep your enemies closer." That was what I needed to do - get to "know my enemy." Even though I was trapped between the walls of my house much of the time, I was determined to figure out what was happening.

One evening, I finally broke the news to my parents over the phone about my situation. I had waited so long because they lived so far away, and they would feel helpless. When I mentioned the struggles I was going through, they tried to convince me to come back to Poland so they could take care of me. That was the last thing I felt I should do!

My sister, who then lived in Australia, would tell me that I was not calling her enough.

"I'm tired!" I would say.

"You're always tired," she replied.

This was hard for me to deal with; I wanted to be back on my feet, helping others. But the pain increased to the point that I did not want to talk to anyone.

## ENGULFED IN PAIN

With everyone giving me advice, I learned that I should never give anyone any advice before knowing all the facts of their situation. There is no one cure-all, no one solution; we are all very different. Even today, I am extremely cautious before I give someone advice.
I finally decided I wouldn't talk to anyone. When the phone rang, I let the answering machine pick up. Engulfed in pain with no help from the medical field, I felt like my life was ending, and I had no control over it.

I barely made it through my 10 to 5 workday, being pleasant to people, painting a smile on my face. In reality, I did not want to be around or talk to anyone.

I no longer had a social life and was losing friendships. This hurt me the most. As a "people person," I was dying inside. I felt useless, without purpose. Depression started to creep in and I no longer felt like I was needed. I felt rejected, even though no one rejected me. On the contrary, I rejected so many invitations and social gatherings that, after a while no one even bothered to ask me.

## "THIS CAN NOT BE NORMAL!"

The pain increased the most when I had my menstrual cycle. Weak, tired, nauseated, I had to stay home in bed for the entire week. It was like this ever since I was a young girl. However, everyone told me that it was normal. I was told that this was part of being a woman and I had to live with it.

Finally, one day I told a girlfriend over dinner, "This cannot be normal." "Well, I must say that I've never heard of anyone suffering quite like you do," she replied.

Over the next week and months, I started reading articles and blogs, trying to figure out answers for my symptoms. My mindset was simple: when you have pain that means you have a problem. While searching and studying, I knew something had to change. Too many times I would be home alone, and become ill or faint. The fainting spells grew to the point that I passed out while working at the retail store. I scared everyone because they did not know what was wrong with me or what to do. I had to stay with some friends for the next three days so I could have supervision to make sure that I would be okay.

I spent the next four years researching and studying, and experimenting with my own body. Winton Churchill's words were very appealing to me, "If you are going through hell, keep going." I continued to see doctors, but there were no results from either conventional or alternative medicines. I was placed on painkillers but they did not help.

In hindsight, I should have looked beyond the pain itself - and so should have my doctors. The pain was only a flashing light and a signal for other conditions that needed attention. When I was offered morphine, I knew I needed to take over my life, before another enemy took over my life - addiction.

## SOMETHING IN COMMON

About this time, my brother, Peter, who lived in Chicago by then, had a friend with similar symptoms as mine. After calling her, I found out that even though we had never met before, we grew up in the same town in Poland. She was three years older than me. Her parents and my parents were friends some years ago. However, she came to America ten years before me, so I did not recall ever meeting her. We conversed over the phone for some time and realized we had similar symptoms. One experience we shared was particularly disturbing.

My brother's friend shared her life experiences in connection to her pain, and she recommended certain books to read. After a rapid read through them all, I realized the first thing I needed to do was change my diet. I discovered that if your body is constantly weak and tired, then a change in diet was the first step to take. I was so desperate and determined that I gave up things I loved and craved fairly easily. With these adjustments, I started noticing a big difference with how I felt and how I could deal with my pain.

The first source of encouragement was that I had somebody with whom I could identify. It made me feel good because I no longer felt I was alone, and had to deal with my situation by myself. For so long I had no one to talk to, but now I had someone who could relate to me. We continued to share information and things that we had discovered or found. We also tried various foods and supplements, hoping something would relieve our pain. We were experimenting with our body, but in a natural way. Later on, we found out that the two of us had the same health condition - endometriosis.

## ON MY OWN

The friend whom I had so much in common with was told that she had endometriosis. However, I only knew that we had similar symptoms and a similar story. No one told me that I had this disease. One of my doctors did mention this disease to me at one time and I begged her to do any test that seemed necessary no matter how much it cost me. I just wanted answers. I asked her to perform a trans-vaginal ultrasound, which was the only way to diagnose me properly.

It is really not good when a patient tells a doctor what to do and to which test to perform. Nevertheless, I figured I looked crazy anyway, so one more time would not make a huge difference. I saw in her face a little sign of irritation, but just to make me happy she agreed.

Even though the doctor was willing to give me this test, she did not think it was necessary and that I was overreacting to my symptoms. In some ways that is understandable, because when you looked at me on the outside I looked very normal. Outwardly, I showed no signs of sickness or pain. Test after test could not reveal what was wrong with me. So by looking at me, you couldn't tell there was anything wrong and I think that people thought that I was crazy or making it all up.

Inside of me, I felt there was some kind of poison that was eating me up, stealing my life, and destroying my body. Other people could not see my pain. They could only see me. Yet, because I was always smiling, had a positive attitude and dressed nice I looked normal.

The people at work never thought there was anything wrong with me until I started fainting. Because I was so good at sales, it appeared that my illness was not hindering my work. Physically, I looked the same each day. Only I knew how much I struggled and how difficult it was for me to deal with life on a day-to-day basis. I did not know how to describe my feelings and symptoms. I did not know how to talk about them, nor know how to make myself more approachable to help others understand my struggles.

## THE PROBLEM WAS NOT KNOWING

At the time, I had no idea how serious my disease was, nor did I know of the countless other women and young girls who were and are infected with this disease. Some people withdraw and others scream for help until they get the right attention. Too many women and young girls are struggling to deal with this disease, not knowing what is attacking their body. But pain should never be taken lightly. It should never be an accepted as a part of life, but ruthlessly dealt with until the right solution is found.

## EPIDEMIC PROPORTIONS

With today's knowledge, there is a ground swell in the medical community to have every woman tested for endometriosis. I believe this is a milestone in the battle against endometriosis. In our society—and the world in general—this disease has reached epidemic proportions, yet still remains so hard to diagnose, and so often misdiagnosed.

How many women and young girls have dealt with pain, especially during their menstrual cycle, and have been told, as I was, "You just have to learn to deal with it"? No! This is not something you have to accept! It is a violation to experience such horrific pain and expect to just deal with it. Why would any female accept something that is robbing her from her ability to be happy?

When you are dealing with agonizing pain, you are giving up your quality of life. You are giving up your happiness. You are giving up your social life. Nevertheless, you are still without answers and have to face your depression. Depression will eventually kill your mind. It will rob your soul. When your mind is not there, you are not here. What a waste of life. When you are talented, when you have gifts, when people see that you have so much to share and to offer, but you continually suffer, that is such a waste of life - for you and for those you love.

If endometriosis can be healed, we could contribute so much more to society. We could help countless women and young girls who are being robbed because they do not have answers to their pain. It is not fair to tell someone to "just deal with what you have." If you are not comfortable with the way you feel, then you don't feel normal. I believe it is very irresponsible for people to allow others to tell them to "just get over it." It is unfair to tell a small girl to just go to sleep, hoping that after she awakens she will feel better.

Another thing: it is not okay to tell a woman she cannot have children just because she has endometriosis. How many endo-babies do we now have in the world? ? Many!

Health practitioners have more academic knowledge, but this health condition remains unknown, hence, advice, direction, and diagnosis for a woman's condition should be given with utmost care and forethought. On the other hand, a woman should never give up, nor should she be scared to take things in her own hands. It is all about belief and self-empowerment.

Winston Churchill said, "Kites rise highest against the wind, not with it." You must believe that you can conquer whatever you are struggling with. Your belief, your mindset, and your will can take you to unbelievable places. By persevering through pain and tribulations, we can find the answers we seek.

*I never stopped looking for answers. And I am glad I never stopped.*

I am glad I did not take my pain for granted. I refused to agree with anything but to become normal. I am happy that I took the steps necessary. Today, I continue to take charge of my life and to seek the answers I need - in every area of my life.

## THE FIRST STEP

I'm sure you want to know what I discovered and how I've turned my life around? I'll get into these things in more detail in later chapters, but for now, changing my diet was the first step towards helping myself. The first thing I needed to do was to get rid of all foods that had toxins. Even though I was reading books directed towards cancer care, I could apply many of the things that were recommended. It was a major and drastic change! I needed to do the extreme, starting with organic foods. Immediately I went to my pantry and refrigerator, and I removed every food item that I thought was unhealthy. I stopped eating meat, choosing instead only fruits, vegetables, and fish. As the pain began to lessen, I had hope, and I knew that it was just a matter of time until I would find my answers. I also knew the only way to optimize my life was to flip it upside down, and I was ready to do it.

I read one book, *The Cure for All Diseases*, by Dr. Hulda Clark, which talked about cleansing. I wondered if it would it work for me? One thing I can tell you is that you will never know how bad you are until you start cleansing. What I have seen and experienced was beyond my imagination. You do not pay enough attention to what we eat. For example, when consuming an apple that looks so good and juicy, do we even think about why it is so *perfectly* round and colorful? Genetic modification, sprays, and pesticides are the reason. So the apple a day that needs to keep the doctor away may not be exactly the apple we talk about.

Such simple activity as eating, which should be a pleasure, was becoming a hard and a difficult thing to accomplish. Going grocery shopping was a serious project; not only did I need a shopping list, but I had to be armed with the right education to make real choices that would affect my health. As I shopped, I felt great sympathy for the mother, who needs to take care of her whole family. Shopping becomes an enterprise!

## FINDING HEALING

Your struggle is something you cannot ignore. It is important to talk about it, to share it. If you suffer with pain as I did, you owe it to yourself to find solutions, not just in "pill form" but solutions that bring healing.

# CHAPTER 3 | What is Endometriosis?

Before we go on, I want to talk a little bit about endometriosis. I had never heard of it before I learned I had it. It wasn't something we talked about in school, even at university. It was a big mystery to me and it may be a mystery to you.

While there are some mysterious things about the disease, there is a lot we can know—and need to know—in order to find a way out of our suffering.

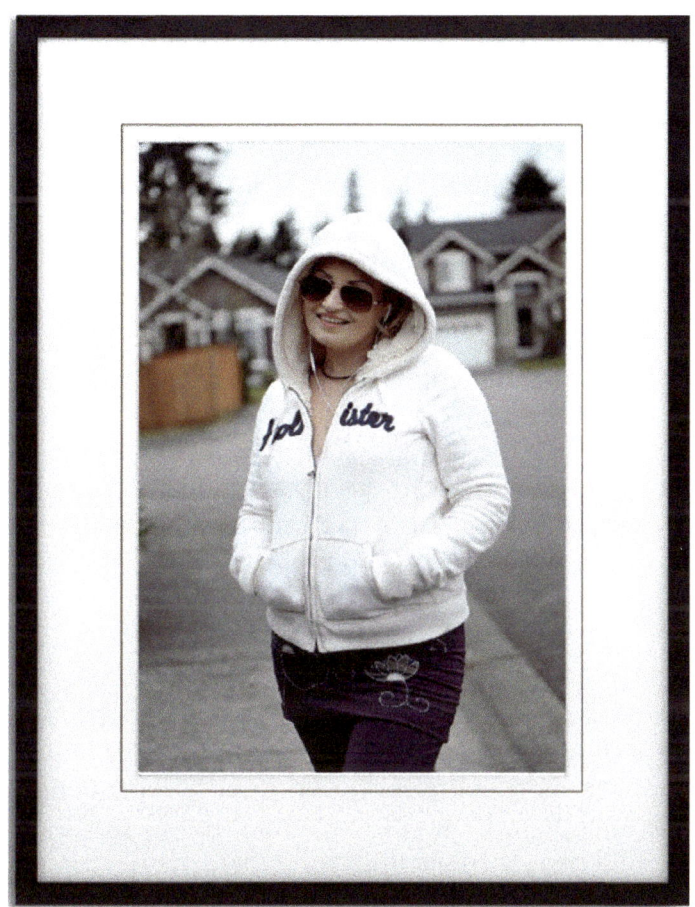

## A PAINFUL DISORDER

According to the Mayo Clinic, endometriosis is an "often painful disorder in which tissue that normally lines the inside of your uterus – the endometrium – grows outside your uterus (endometrial implant). Endometriosis most commonly involves your ovaries, bowel, or the tissue lining your pelvis. Rarely, endometrial tissue may spread beyond your pelvic region. In endometriosis, displaced endometrial tissue continues to act as it normally would – it thickens, breaks down and bleeds with each menstrual cycle. Because this displaced tissue has no way to exit your body, it becomes trapped. When endometriosis involves the ovaries, cysts called endometriomas may form. Surrounding tissue can become irritated, eventually developing scar tissue and adhesions – abnormal tissue that binds organs together. Endometriosis can cause pain – sometimes severe – especially during your period. Fertility problems also may develop. Fortunately, effective treatments are available."[2]

## LIFE-DAMAGING CONDITION

That definition says that endometriosis is, but it doesn't begin to cover what endometriosis does to a woman, to her self-image, to her relationships, to her life. Endometriosis is not only a gynecological problem; it affects all areas of your body, including your kidney or bladder, because the cells are continuously growing outside your uterus. It may not be a *life-threatening* condition but it is a *life-damaging* condition.

Endometriosis has many faces. It has symptoms that may be assigned to many other diseases or health conditions. The cells can grow just about everywhere outside the uterus and cause problems in various areas in your body. It can cause deep pelvic pain, and lower abdominal pain. It can be accompanied by bowel and bladder symptoms. The pain is really unpredictable.

Symptoms of endometriosis may include one or more of the following:

- Chronic or intermittent pelvic pain
- Dysmenorrhea (painful menstruation)
- Infertility
- Painful sexual intercourse
- Painful bowel movements
- Fatigue
- Heavy or irregular bleeding
- Pain during ovulation
- Gastrointestinal problems (constipation, diarrhea, bloating)
- Painful urination
- Lower back pain

---

[2] http://www.mayoclinic.org/diseases-conditions/endometriosis/basics/definition/con-20013968

## UNKNOWN CAUSES

No one really knows what causes endometriosis. According to American Pregnancy, one possible cause of endometriosis is menstrual tissue that backs up during menstruation. Another theory is that it is a genetic birth abnormality caused when endometrial cells develop outside the uterus. Yet another theory says that it is hereditary since women with a family history of the disease are more apt to develop it themselves.

## CHERNOBYL

I don't know for sure what caused me to have endometriosis. I now know that my grandmother probably had it—and endometriosis runs in families. However, I do think that it is linked to that fateful day in April 1986 when I was exposed to radiation from Chernobyl.

The nuclear accident at Chernobyl is one of the two worst nuclear diasters in the world. Only it and the Fukushima Daiichi nuclear disaster in 2011 have the maximum classifications on the International Nuclear Event Scale.

The nuclear power station located in the Ukraine contained four nuclear reactors. On April 26, 1986, during a test, an explosion occurred that melted the fuel rods, ignited the reactor's covering, and released a cloud of radiation that blanketed Europe, including my native Poland. Although only a handful of people died shortly after the disaser, "The Belarus National Academy of Sciences estimates 270,000 people in the region around the accident site will develop cancer as a result of Chernobyl radiation and that 93,000 of those cases are likely to be fatal."[3]

While endometriosis isn't cancer, it is an abnormality in a woman's reproductive system—and authorities know that the reproductive system is one of the most sensitive to things like environmental toxins and radiation.

I may never be able to prove that my endometriosis was directly caused by the radiation from Chernobyl, but in my heart I know that

---

[3] http://environment.about.com/od/chernobyl/p/chernobyl.htm

it had to have had an effect.

The day I came home after the "plant accident," my family had taken Lugol, a type of iodine used to help prevent the effects of radiation poisoning. With Russian denial of any possible danger from the "accident" at Chernobyl, the Polish government decided it was mandatory for the benefit of its citizens and especially children to take caution. The government said that we were not to panic, but, unbeknownst to the general population, a decision was made to assume the worst-case scenario—that we had been exposed to deadly and damaging radiation.

Over the next few years, we didn't think much about that fateful day. We went on with our lives, but it was already too late for many. We soon learned of pregnant women suffering from miscarriages or delivering dead babies. Who would take the blame? Certainly not the government.

My aunt, who was pregnant with twins, was given Lugol that April. On December 28 I remember the phone rang, and we were all anticipating the birth of two beautiful babies. And yes they were born - stillborn! December 28 will live in infamy in my mind; my grandpa was born on that same date and I was hoping to have two more cousins. Worse, twenty years later my aunt started feeling extremely sick for no apparent reason. Finally, she was diagnosed with a very rare leukemia, something that had never been found in our family history. Two days after the diagnosis, she passed away. Nobody recalled or even mentioned Chernobyl.

The Chernobyl fallout was invisible, which caused people not to believe it!

*Radiation cannot be seen, but it had definitely saturated our environment. It was and is a silent killer, and a deformer of life, both physical and mental.*

That April day in 1986 changed my life entirely and the lives of many others. But as we move on, we forget things. We face different challenges and embark on new discoveries. We do not realize that what we struggle with today could very well be the result of something that happened years ago.

## CONNECTING THE DOTS

It took me a long time to realize to connect the dots. The Soviets were manipulating the numbers of radiation poisoning victims and death rates so it was very difficult to estimate and evaluate. The lies could reveal so many more answers if the truth were told. But in Poland and all Eastern Bloc countries, people preferred to live in denial, with the governments leading the way. Would anyone in Poland connect Chernobyl to the fact that, twenty years later, there was an epidemic of thyroid cancer? It is sad that people who were trying to disclose facts on Chernobyl were silenced, removed, or simply did not "make it."

However, as I began to search for answers to my pain, I began to put the pieces of the puzzle together.

It was all really simple. The area of Chernobyl remains uninhabitable. For twenty plus years, we had lived with radioactive food that continues to contaminate the Polish population. No global statistics have yet been made public. There was, however, a doctor who was working on illnesses among the population in the contaminated area, who published his findings in 1996. His writings were immediately condemned by the government, and he was arrested for corruption and sentenced to five years in prison.

Sadly today, Chernobyl and its lessons seem to be fading into memory. Yet the people of Poland and all Eastern Bloc countries have no clear information. Here is another lesson I've learned: we are told we live in a free world, with freedom of speech, the right to believe and the choice to choose our own lives. But if we allow those in power to usurp these, not only do we suffer, but our children will reap the consequences of our inaction.

In the end, however, why and how I got this life-alterning disease isn't as important as the fact that I have learned how to live a full and rewarding life despite it.

And that is what I want to share with you.

# CHAPTER 4
# Misconceptions and Myths

One of the most important things to understand is there is a solution for every problem. This is not very easy to accept, especially if you are a woman. While men fix things, when women talk about our problems, we do not necessarily look for answers. It is simply not in our nature.

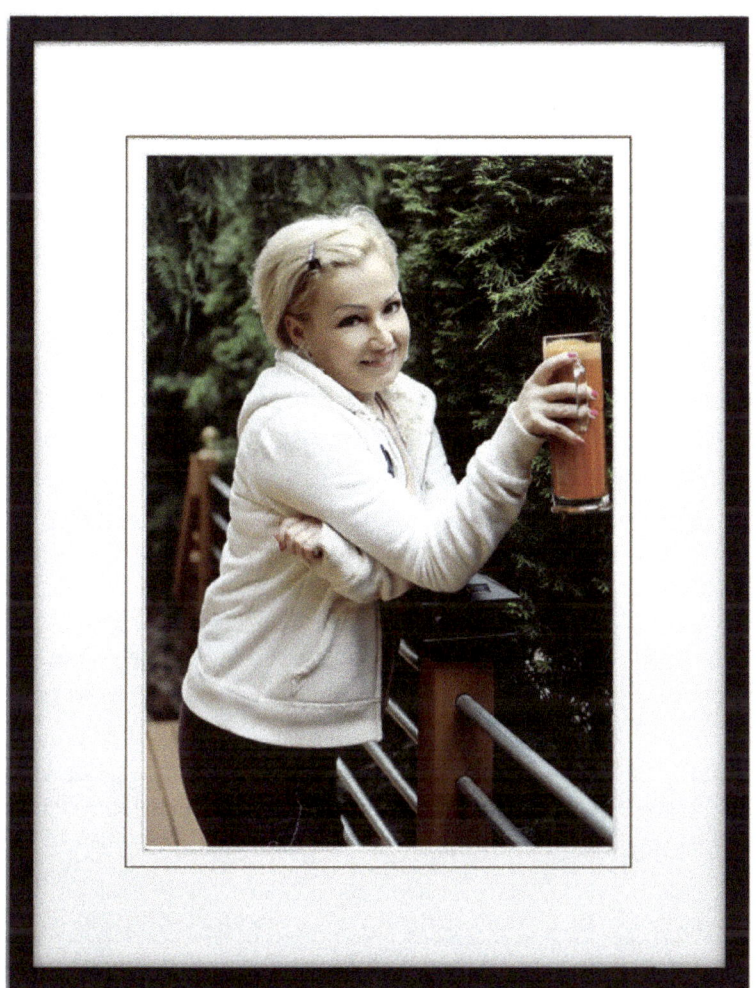

## RECOGNIZING THE SOURCE OF DISEASE

One of the factors when dealing with endometriosis is recognizing the source behind the disease. We must recognize that what is environmental cannot be treated with conventional means. Conventional medicine attempts to treat the condition, symptoms, and the disease with unnatural supplements. To treat this disease properly, it must be treated naturally. The answer is not hormonal treatment. Each woman has a different hormonal level and so one treatment cannot help a woman because each one is different. For instance, some women have excess bleeding and some do not. Some can exercise and some cannot. Scientific experiments with mice and rats have proven that certain foods can cause endometriosis.

So I encourage women to understand that what they eat can affect their body. I say to every woman and to everybody to not eat manufactured foods. In order for us to understand more, I encourage people to realize that things will not change overnight, but by having the right knowledge you will see drastic changes over time. If you suffer from any health condition for many years, and in the meantime you have been misdiagnosed and mistreated to reverse all these, you need to take into consideration that it may take an equal amount of time for recovery. Our body regenerates over time. Expecting instant solutions will only bring disappointments.

When sharing with people who suffer from this disease, I explain the importance of eating right but some refuse to listen. Perhaps, because we take the importance of food too lightly. To make a point I will bring up the car example. We will not argue with the car manufacturer's factory recommendation to put water or gas, in our gas tank right? Even if it would save us lots of money we still know water will never feed the engine, and if we decide to go against these recommendations we would not go far. Nutrition is a fuel to your body and malnutrition will only keep it going for so long.

As much as doctors are working hard to find the solution at this point while trying to help you, they still experiment and try and learn, just like you.

## LISTEN TO YOUR BODY

If this is the case then how can one criticize you if you choose to change your diet as a cure? Many of the experiments on women and young girls today are doing more damage than good. My suggestion is listen to your body get into your rhythm and try to understand it. Nobody will understand your body as well as you do. When it comes to food, your body will tell you what is good for you and what is not. For instance when your body tells you that you are tired, do not force yourself to keep going. You need to be very conscious of all areas of your body. Do not ignore any symptoms because the smallest can be very important. Your body is always talking to you, ignoring the inner voice will come back to you at some point and very often times it is late or even too late, do not let this happen. Take your time and pay attention. Do not run too quickly through your life. Your body is not a mobile device as you may think, we cant upgrade every few months, you have your body once and forever, so take good care of it.

We should be open-minded to whatever solutions may present themselves. I am not saying to never go to a medical doctor. But what I am saying is to attempt a nonconventional treatment. I went to many doctors, but I chose to choose what my body chose for me. I had to make major adjustments to cleanse my body. I used to work out three times a week kickboxing, swimming, etc. I tried to exercise I was told it was supposed to be good for me and would make me feel better. Actually, the exercise was pushing my body to its limits and doing more harm than good. So I stopped. I started feeling better. I exercise today but then I needed to give my body a break.

Sometimes you will exercise more and sometimes you will exercise less. Your body goes to different intervals; learn how to listen to your bodies signals and what is telling you. Trust your intuition and just go with it.

Summarizing the point: if something appears to be your solution, take it no matter from which source it comes.

### NEVER GIVE UP

Do not give up. It will not last forever. My life became extraordinary and I believe that yours can too. I believe I can show you how to cope with your issues gracefully. Unless you keep things in balance, you will not feel good no matter what you suffer from. You need to balance everything.

If you can find a good nutritionist, you can bring a balance to your body. Over time, you can learn to function properly. Be prepared for constant changes and intervals in your lifestyle. If something is good for you now, it may become not good later. If some medications work for you now, you may need to change them later. As hard as change is, it is good for you. If someone will tell you to eat cabbage because it is good for you, it doesn't mean you have to eat it three times a day for the rest of your life. There are different things there that are good for you. Your body also gets used to medication and foods and it needs change. Take it as an attribute not a challenge. It will only make your life more interesting not boring. We cannot change all the pollution that is around us and all the toxic foods, but we can do the right things that can make us feel better. Support is what comes to my mind. Support the best you can, with whatever you can. If you know for a fact this is something you will live with forever, instead of turning this into disaster, support yourself. You can only do as much as you can do with what you have. This way you will develop the ability to look at things with a broader perspective and without panicking and getting anxious. Set your mind on the mountain that will take you through obstacles that are going to be everyday present in your life, regardless of endometriosis. You CAN do it!

## YOU ARE VALUABLE

I want to share with you my experience and my knowledge and my secrets that have made my life so enjoyable. We may have this disease, but we can live on our own beach and life can be wonderful. Do not feel isolated. You are valuable; never more so than when you open up and share. There is light at the end of the tunnel. You are not alone. You may become a good leader to help another woman find the light at the end of the tunnel.

I am not an endocrinologist or gynecologist. But as a psychologist, I understand that each of us has to develop our own path -and that takes huge determination and persistence. But If you are willing to satisfy your curiosity, become knowledgeable, and take the journey, life with endometriosis can be fulfilling, satisfying, and even enjoyable. You know YOU can help so many women, but FIRST you must help yourself. I cannot heal you completely because I am not completely healed myself. However, I manage my disease and you can manage yours. I know how to deal with my pain. I know what to expect. I know how to respond to it, and so can you. I know there is no one cure that will heal everyone. There is no one treatment. We are all different individuals and there is only one of you.

You cannot find an instant remedy. There is no such thing. We see a tendency to go back to grandma style for living healthy. We look for solutions thinking they must be complicated as they are unknown, however such things aren't as complicated as they first appear–they are actually very simple. Simple life, simple food–everything totally simplified. Living our "sophisticated" lives we thoughtlessly fueled our body with things that now need to be withdrawn. How ironic. We cannot expect that we can continue to damage and pollute our body with manufactured foods. We need to detox our bodies and cleanse it. Think of yourself as a filter, filter for all around you: air, food, stress. You take it all, and you need support the filtering because your body was not build to function in such polluted environment. We need to turn on all the lights so the shadow is gone and we become strong. You need to fell healthy and be free. You can become your very own master. Share your pain until you will not have it.

In my case, I needed to go beyond my natural inclination of "getting it off my shoulders." That simply was not enough.

## ACKNOWLEDGING FEELINGS

One day, while drinking tea and honey with my grandmother, who had come over from Poland to visit me, she noticed that I was not feeling well. She wanted to know why I was suddenly showing signs of depression. I explained how I felt, and that after going to doctors, I believed that I had a disease called endometriosis. As my grandmother listened, she simply smiled and nodded her head. I knew that she loved me so I was somewhat surprised that after describing my symptoms, she took it so lightly. In some ways, it was if I was ignored. For me it was something very important and I thought she did not know how to respond.

Then, surprisingly, she told me that she could relate to everything I just told her. While raising two children, she learned to "press" her way through her pain. She did not know why she suffered from agonizing pain, because nobody talked about it at that time.

When a newborn cries, someone comes to its rescue. No one serves a baby drugs to keep it quiet. No one leaves it in a crib and waits until the crying stops. On the contrary, everyone is concerned, trying to find a way to figure out what is wrong. No one assumes that the baby is crazy, insane, or it is "only in your (the baby's) head."

In my situation, no one bothered to look beyond my symptoms to find out what was wrong with me. No one really tried to understand why I was having such difficulties and experiencing so much pain.

I felt like a crying baby only no one was there to hold me or to give me pacifier nor to rum my belly. I was a baby that needed to grow up fast and take over her life and make it better.

## ANOTHER STORY

I know someone who is a couple of years older than me who was also diagnosed with endometriosis. Her sickness affected her marriage tremendously. Unfortunately, she did not have a supportive husband while she was going through her illness. His ultimate goal was to have children, but she could not get pregnant. He attempted to force her to go under hormonal treatment and surgeries because all he cared about what her getting pregnant. When she was unable to conceive, he considered her an unproductive product. For him she was simply defective, like anything else that was broken. I dare to say his poor approach came from his upbringing where a woman's duty was at home, in the kitchen, and with children. He chose to cultivate this upbringing, and strongly believed he was doing the right thing. It was a little how we were taught in our Polish society. I was taught that having sex was like having your menstrual cycle, it was not pleasurable; it was for more for procreation, not pleasure.

Unfortunately, my friend's husband had insufficient knowledge of this disease. She continued to have excruciating pain and high medical bills, both of which were destroying their relationship. He did not go with her to the doctor visits, nor did he offer help of any kind. She was dealing with extreme pain, which eventually made her feel unattractive. She became depressed because she could not get pregnant or make her husband happy.

Besides her pain and unhappiness, she had to deal with her husband, who was very impatient and was getting more and more irritated, because he was constantly unhappy and made her feel like it was her fault. Her health problems, and the deteriorating relationship, killed the marriage. Because she could not get any sympathy from him, she turned to others who cared more about her and her condition. Eventually her parents came to stay with her because it was common for her to pass out and have to be taken to the hospital by ambulance. But even though they cared so much, her pain was beyond their expertise. They did not know how to help her. Her husband moved on and they divorced.

Of course, it is very sad their relationship ended, but it is far more sad that a woman can feel guilty for being sick and because she cannot deliver a child. Would we ever make our children feel guilty because they have the flu or cancer? How crazy does it sound? Yet many women with endometriosis feel guilty since they cannot deliver a baby.

## EXPECTATIONS

This disease has an extreme influence upon how a woman feels about herself. She feels like a broken element; incomplete as a person. My grandmother is a great example. She was a strong woman who suffered silently. Nevertheless, this is not what a woman wants to be praised for. Medals are not given for enduring pain gracefully. Because she was not treated right, eventually my grandmother needed to undergo a hysterectomy. People didn't think it was such a big deal. She had served her duty as a woman by delivering two babies.

Going alone with my care examples, here is another one. When you have a flat tire you do not remove it and ride only in three wheels, you fix it, replace it and continue your trip. It almost shows that cars are being taken better care of. Some will say that hysterectomy actually made them feel better, and I believe, but only because it was a fast remedy that was actually a failure to provide the 'repair' solution.

It is sad to say but this is how it goes: when you are still in a reproductive age, there are "expectations" of you. Once you pass this age, and you need to have all things removed, well, that is not such a great loss. How ironic! It is almost like saying to a soccer player after he retires that he will not need his legs anymore, so he should simply get them amputated.

Why would we make a hasty decision to remove organs that are integral part of a woman body? Why should we interrupt the natural functioning of our bodies?

## SOME FACTS AND FIGURES

Endometriosis has existed for a long time. There is no age bracket for this disease. You can be a young girl or an older woman. It does not matter whether you have had a baby or after menopause, this disease attacks any woman. It is growing common these days with teenage girls. The average woman is 27 when she is first diagnosed with endometriosis. Most women suffer with pain—and have symptoms—up to a full decade prior to diagnosis. Approximately 176 million women and girls worldwide suffer from endometriosis; 8.5 million in North America alone. [4] Today, it is considered as a major unrecognized disease worldwide. Costs for diagnosis in 2012 in the US reached $69 billion. [5] It is a similar economic burden to diabetes, Crohn's disease, and rheumatoid arthritis.

Unfortunately, it can take a lifetime to detect this disease because many of the symptoms can remain hidden and undetected, and many take years to be properly diagnosed. Worse, severe endometriosis may have few symptoms!

---

[4] http://www.endofound.org/endometriosis

[5] http://humrep.oxfordjournals.org/content/early/2012/03/14/humrep.des073.full.pdf

## LOOKING FOR HELP

While you looking for solutions and answers, and optimizing your health, and even while fighting endometriosis, you end up going to many doctors. I have seen several gynecologists, oncologists, gone to pain clinics, and finally a psychologist. Instead of diagnosing the disease, I was told I had mental challenges. It is much easier to diagnose someone as "crazy" than to find answers to their sickness. I was told that the headaches, migraines, cramps, and pain were not cancer, so it must be "all in your head."

Going to see doctors becomes a normal routine in your life. And you are constantly diagnosed with many other conditions. They check your stomach, say nothing is wrong, so they send you to another doctor for your intestines...it goes on and on. Although your bladder may be in pain, it is not the problem. There are endless trips to the hospital, to the doctors, to the specialist, but you do not get better. I saw so many doctors, needles, and exams--not to mention the difficulties with bowel movements and the menstrual cycle.

Eventually your body wears down and you become unemployable, because you are having surgeries, or you are in recovery, or you have too many visits to the doctor. You end up going to the doctor more than you would go to a movie theater. Who would want to hire someone like that? If you are not working for a family member or a close friend, you will probably not keep that job very long.

I understand. As I was learning about my disease, I needed people who would support me and help me along the way. I could have never made it without these kinds of people. I was fortunate enough to have people in my life who did not simply cut me off. I cannot tell you how lucky I was and how grateful I am today to all those who never let me feel left alone, never left behind, and never thought I was crazy. I have worked with the nicest and most compassionate people who, despite of not knowing and understanding what was going on with me, have always been there for me without any pre-conceived assumptions.

## TALKING ABOUT THE TABOO

I know many girls and women who lose hope because they do not know enough about endometriosis. I believe that it is important that we talk about this, even though it is unpopular and for many, it is still a taboo. Countless women suffer from it. We cannot just put our head in the sand and pretend as if it is not there. It affects a woman physically emotionally, and their entire well-being. There were so many days that I just laid in bed and could not do anything. I was so weak in my body that I could not even do normal housecleaning. It became physically and mentally overwhelming.

To you who are reading this book, I want to encourage you: It is really up to you how much you are willing to talk about it. The more we talk, the more we know. The more doors we knock on, the more open up. We need to realize that each and every case is individual, so we must break the ice and pour our pain out.

## MISCONCEPTIONS AND MYTHS

There are many misconceptions and myths about this disease. For example, a young girl who is in her menstrual cycle is told she is too young to have the disease. Or that she cannot have children, or that pregnancy will heal her, or that laparoscopy will definitely help her. The truth is, all these answers can be correct, and all of them can be completely wrong, depending on the case we are dealing with.

There is so much misunderstanding about infertility, pregnancy, and emotional conditions. A woman with this disease begins to suffer two weeks before her period. She gets tired and weary. After her period she continues to bleed, leaving only two weeks out of the month to catch up on life. Every person who suffers with this disease must be treated as an individual, because symptoms vary with each person. Because there are so many conditions and different types of symptoms, many times it is very difficult to diagnose. Therefore, we need to be educated, be more open about the topic, and be willing to talk about it, without shame or being embarrassed.

Because it is considered a "woman's disease," it is overlooked many times and considered to be "part of being a female." We are simply told it is just something we must live with, but that is not the case. It is not ok to be sick period, gender doesn't matter and age doesn't matter. It is simply not ok. Being companionate and empathetic very often is a medicine itself.

## FAMOUS SUFFERERS

### Whoopi Goldberg

Very famous and important women suffer with this disease as well. For example, Whoopi Goldberg is an American comedian, actress, singer-songwriter, political activist, author, and talk show host. She found out she had endometriosis in the 70s. She has one daughter, Alexandria, born in 1973.

### Padma Lakshmi

Padma Lakshmi is an Indian American author, actress, model, and television presenter. She also co-founded the Endometriosis Foundation of America. Padma suffered with pain for more than twenty years and was told it was "all in her head" before she was correctly diagnosed. While having surgery, it was revealed she had two cysts on each of her ovaries and was put on birth control. She gave birth to her daughter, Krishna, in 2010.

### Julianne Hough

Julianne Hough is an American professional ballroom dancer, singer, and actress. She was starring in Dancing with the Stars in 2008 when she knew her body had taken all it could. She was in agony but ignored producers' pleas to go to the hospital.

The next morning Julianne had an ultrasound, which revealed she had a cyst on her left ovary and a lot of scar tissue outside of her uterus, which had spread to her appendix and right hip. She had laparoscopic surgery a week later, forcing her to leave the show mid-season. The endometriosis had also spread to her Fallopian tubes and bladder. Julianne believes she started suffering with pain from the disease around 2003. Her mother and sister also have endometriosis.

American actress, Susan Sarandon, was diagnosed with endometriosis in 1983, after suffering from pain, irregular bleeding, and fainting. She was told that if she ever wanted children she would have to have surgery, and was put on birth control pills and painkillers. Today, she has three children, a daughter, Eva, born in 1985 and two sons, Jack, born in 1989, and Miles, born in 1992.

The world-famous Marylyn Monroe, an American actress, model and singer, died at age 36. She never had children though she was pregnant numerous times. All of her pregnancies ended in miscarriage and, reportedly, at least one ectopic pregnancy due to her severe endometriosis. Rumors say she went into one surgery with a note taped to her stomach, pleading with the doctors not to remove her reproductive organs. Although there is much mystery surrounding her death, many think it is indirectly linked to her endometriosis. The disease caused her to become addicted to painkillers, which in turn aggravated her psychological problems. Her X-rays from one of her surgeries for the disease sold for $54,000 at auction[6]

## NOT JUST A FEMALE PROBLEM

This book is not just for women who suffer with this disease. It is for both men and women alike, because it is about mutual understanding and mutual support. It is about having open communication and learning how to deal with the disease, learning how to fight it, and conquer it. It is important for men to understand what a woman is going through, otherwise, he will accuse her of making excuses about migraines, tiredness, and weakness as an excuse not to have sexual intercourse.

---

[6]http://emlwy.blogspot.com/2013/04/celebrities-with-endometriosis.html

A man must learn more about this disease so he can look beyond his companion, and become compassionate and understanding to what she is going through.

If you are uneducated, you will ignore the warning signs and not realize how serious this disease can be. Once you understand what the disease is and how to fight it, men and women can combine their strengths and weaknesses to carry each other through it. However, finding more information can be a difficult thing.

Knowledge will very likely save relationship and will strengthen them. There is nothing worse then expecting from someone something one cannot deliver simply because he is not aware of it. If your partner will know why you need to stay in bed for a week or as long as you need to stay, then it won't cause a problem. If your partner knows it makes a difference.

# CHAPTER 5 | Fertility Issues

One of the major problems that arise with endometriosis is the question of fertility. If you have endometriosis, you have probably wondered, "Can this disease affect my ability to get pregnant?" There is a large body of evidence that demonstrates an association between endometriosis and infertility. The reality is that endometriosis makes it more difficult to get pregnant and is one of the top three causes of female infertility. Endometriosis can be found in up to 50% of infertile women.[7] Studies find that about 21% to 44% of infertile women have endometriosis, but only 4% to 22% of fertile women. Infertility patients with untreated mild endometriosis conceive on their own at a rate of 2% to 4.5% per month, compared to a 15% to 20% monthly fertility rate in normal couples. Infertility patients with moderate and severe endometriosis have monthly pregnancy rates of less than 2%.[8] While it is one of the most treatable causes of infertility, it remains the least treated.[9]

---

[7] http://www.healthywomen.org/content/article/endometriosis-and-pregnancy
[8] www.asrm.org/Endometriosis_booklet/
[9] www.endofound.org/endometriosis

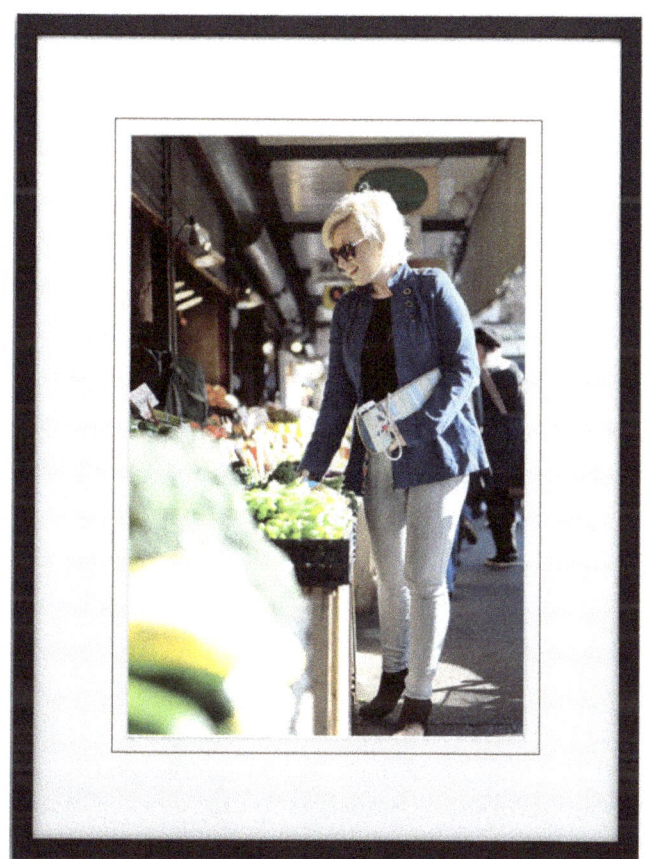

Even though endometriosis is associated strongly with infertility, not all women who have endometriosis are infertile. For example, many women undergoing tubal sterilization procedures are noted to have endometriosis.

As we have said before, endometriosis is a condition where endometrial tissue grows outside the uterus, causing pockets of tissue to build up in and around the Fallopian tubes, ovaries, bladder, and other parts of the pelvic area. Mild endometriosis can have a direct effect on a woman's ability to get pregnant due to the increased chance of adhesion growth in the ovaries, hindering the implantation process of the egg in the uterus. According to an article on Endometriosis.org, women with endometriosis may also have a higher risk of miscarriages.

It is presumed that endometriosis alters the pelvic environment in a number of subtle but important ways. Theories include inflammation, altered immune system, hormonal changes, abnormal function of the Fallopian tube, or impaired fertilization and implantation. It is easier to understand how moderate or severe endometriosis reduces fertility, since major pelvic adhesions, when present, may prevent the release of eggs, block sperm entry into the Fallopian tube, and prevent the Fallopian tubes' ability to pick up eggs during ovulation. [10]

One theory that is getting a lot of attention suggests endometriosis may be related to an underlying immune condition that increases inflammation. Chemicals called cytokines, released when the immune system sweeps in to fix a problem, cause inflammation, in part. Endometrial tissue outside the uterus is certainly one of those problems! In addition, studies find higher levels of cytokines in the fluid within the peritoneum, which encloses the gastrointestinal and reproductive organs.

Other studies suggest that high levels of cytokines can negatively affect not only fertility, but also the outcome of pregnancy and the health of embryos. Cytokines can also affect the health of your eggs, with studies finding that women with endometriosis have more problems related to their ability to produce healthy eggs than those without the disease. Unhealthy eggs are much less likely to lead to a pregnancy even if a sperm reaches them.

When implantation occurs, the endometrial tissue secretes important hormones into the uterus in order to prepare it for pregnancy. When the endometrial tissue has built up outside the uterus, the secretions have nowhere to go, and often are passed through the abdominal cavity instead of the uterus. These misplaced hormones will cause the body to become confused, and allow the woman to continue to ovulate even though pregnancy has already occurred. When ovulation continues, the body will go through its normal process of wanting to shed its old lining (including the fertilized egg) causing a very early miscarriage.

---

[10] www.asrm.org/Endometriosis_booklet/

Despite potential complications, many women with endometriosis can conceive and have successful pregnancies. Conception can happen without intervention for about half of the women with endometriosis. However, if the symptoms are severe, a number of treatments that will increase a woman's chances of conception.

## A PROGRESSIVE DISEASE

Endometriosis is a progressive disease, and its damaging effects can become more severe over time. For this reason, women suffering from endometriosis who wish to become pregnant are encouraged not to put off efforts to conceive. Such was the case with me when the doctor told me I only had a three-month window to get pregnant, or accept the fact I would never have children.

When diagnosed with endometriosis, the amount, and location of the disease determines whether it has considered minimal, mild, moderate, or severe. In more severe cases, scar tissue from endometriosis adheres to the ovaries or Fallopian tubes, and egg release may be restricted or blocked, making fertilization difficult or impossible. Blood-filled cysts called endometriomas can develop and compress the ovaries, which can damage egg supply or inhibit ovulation.

Women with endometriosis may also produce cells that attack and potentially destroy sperm. Additionally, endometriosis has been linked to an overproduction of prostaglandins, which can interfere with normal reproductive processes. Unsustainable ectopic pregnancies, where a fertilized egg does not move from the Fallopian tube to the uterus, are more common in women with endometriosis. In addition, if a woman with endometriosis experiences pain during intercourse, she may be inclined to have sex less frequently, limiting the possibility of her getting pregnant.

The most common treatment is to have surgery to remove the built-up lining within the pelvic area. Removal of an ovarian endometrioma will allow the egg to be released into the Fallopian tube and travel down to the uterus for fertilization. This type of surgery may also help decrease the pain levels some women experience during ovulation, and help regulate hormone levels within the body. Surgery may also help reproductive specialists to harvest eggs for in vitro fertilization (IVF) if the removal of the extra endometrial tissue is not successful on its own.

## EMOTIONAL ROLLER COASTER

Like all women trying to get pregnant, you have a lot to deal with. You are taking time off from work for doctor appointments, having blood drawn, having pelvic exams, ultrasounds injection, taking basal temperatures, timing intercourse and undergoing various diagnosis procedures. But you also have to deal with being on an emotional roller coaster, a husband who may not participate in your medical treatments as much as you would like, friends and family who make insensitive comments, and social situations that are almost unbearably painful, like a baby shower.

The whirlwind of emotions that infertility brings can feel overwhelming. Sometimes knowing that your feelings are normal can help. You may be grieving over the sense of loss for the child or children you imagined having one day. You may also feel that you are missing the experience of parenthood or the act of having a biological child. You may feel angry at life in general. You may also feel angry or jealous that parenthood seems to come easily to others. You might tell yourself that you just know next month will bring a positive pregnancy test, and then, when it does not, feel a huge sense of sadness and shock.

Some women may feel that a diagnosis of infertility makes them less feminine. You may also feel that you are somehow less of a person if you cannot have a child on your own. You may feel a lack of control, knowing that you can do nothing to guarantee or know if treatments will work.

## RELATIONSHIPS AND FINANCES

Infertility can also put stress on your relationship, with studies showing that couples dealing with infertility are more likely to feel unhappy with themselves and their marriages. Infertility may affect your relationship in a number of ways. The first issue that effects men more than women is sexual tension. Especially around ovulation, sex may feel more like a chore than an enjoyable way to express love for each other. Men may experience performance anxiety, leading to feelings of guilt or shame.

Another tension is the financial stress. Fertility treatment costs can quickly add up. Everything from deciding how much you are willing to pay to coping with the financial strain or debt can create a great deal of stress between couples. Another factor couples deal with is the fear of abandonment, especially for the partner with the infertility diagnosis; she may be afraid that her partner will want to leave her to have children with someone else.

Along with the difficulties coping with endometriosis, when dealing with infertility, too often arguments about treatments arise. Deciding which treatments or options to try, when to stop seeking treatment, or when to take a break can put tremendous strain on a couple.

## DEVELOP COPING SKILLS

With the myriad of feelings surrounding infertility, good coping skills are essential. The first step when attempting to cope is to acknowledge your feelings. Holding everything inside does not help. It actually takes more mental energy to hold your feelings back than to express them. Allow yourself time to feel the sadness, anger, and frustration.

Trying to cope without support is often difficult. I encourage you to seek support, whether through friends, professional counseling, groups or online forums, or finding somewhere to talk with people who understand can help you feel less alone. With the right support, being alone is more manageable. However, being alone can cause loneliness. Make the most of being alone by learning how to relax and calm yourself can help when feelings get intense and during treatments.

During those times when you feel all alone, take time to talk to your partner about your feelings. Keep in mind, though, that men and women cope with stress in different ways. Women are more likely to express their sadness, while men tend to hold things inside. Neither way is wrong, just different.

To cope, learn as much as you can about how endometriosis affects fertility. The more you know about infertility, including alternatives like adoption or living child-free, the more in control you will feel. As hard as it might sound, do not allow infertility to take over your life. It will paralyze you from having a life and developing relationships. If it seems like infertility is all you and your partner talk about together, set a specified time each day for the topic, and use the rest of the day to talk about other things.

### DIFFICULTIES WITH SEX

As I have already mentioned, having endometriosis can make sex difficult, and when you are battling infertility, sex can quickly become more like a chore, rather than a fun way to express love for each other. Try to keep things loving and exciting. Light candles, play fun music, or watch romantic movies, whatever makes you both feel good.

Many couples find that professional individual or couples' counseling can help them cope with the emotional stress of infertility. If you find yourself feeling constantly sad or anxious, not sleeping well or oversleeping, feeling completely isolated, or having thoughts of death and dying, then it is especially important that you speak to your doctor about your feelings.

# CHAPTER 6
# What is a Woman?

In this chapter, I would like to concentrate on the woman who, sometimes when facing problems such as this complex disease, loses herself. She can easily underestimate herself and can lose confidence. She may even forget that others are ready to support her. Like me, she may tend to belittle herself, especially when things are expected of her and she cannot deliver.

I would like to encourage all women to read Why Men Love Bitches . . . From Doormat to Dream Girl - A Woman's Guide to Holding her Own in a Relationship by Sherry Argov. It explains all the stereotypes of a woman and shows how men and women think completely the opposite.

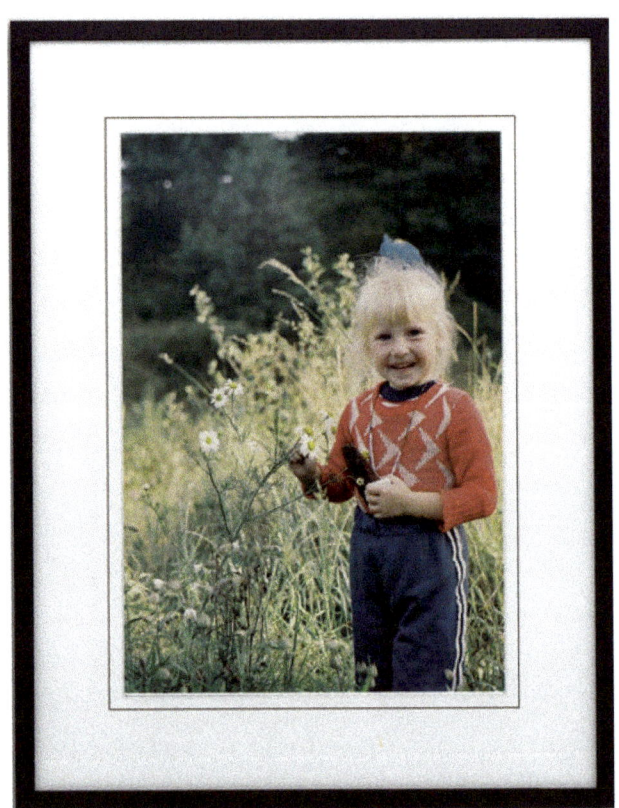

## A WOMAN'S BRAIN

A woman's brain is wired differently from a man's. In fact, a woman's brain is wired like the Internet, and a man's brain consists of square boxes that are organized in a great order. A man is logically-based, focused, and direct, while a woman's brain is emotionally-centered, scattered, and more easily distracted. Ask a man what he thinks after watching an emotionally-charged movie or TV show, and he will say, "It was okay," or "Not bad." Ask a woman what she thinks of the same movie and you will hear every detail, with tears and sniffles for the next 30 to 40 minutes. Neither response is wrong. It is just the way men and women are wired mentally. Men can get easily confused listening to a woman who thinks and talks about totally unrelated subjects in one sentence. That is because, for a woman, changing topics in the middle of a thought fits her natural makeup.

## A WOMAN'S BODY

A woman's body is in a constant state of change due to hormones. A woman can say one thing and then do another. She puts on a dress, only to change two more times. And when she thinks she has the right outfit, she will typically ask her partner, "How does this look?" Then the pressure is on. The response will determine if she changes again, or accepts the outfit she is wearing as suitable for public display. This might come across erratic or irrational to a man, but for a woman everything about her body and her mind is changing.

## A WOMAN'S MOOD

A woman's mood is constantly changing. For instance, if she sees something while riding in the car, she will abruptly change the subject. Simply put, a woman is an emotional being, period.

Talking about how men and women deal with their emotions is like comparing apples to oranges. Although men are emotional creatures, just like women, they do not act or respond in the same manner as a woman. Men tend to be more reclusive when it comes to emotional issues. Most men, when they are irritated, will withdraw. They will walk away from the situation. Some men will even leave the room or the house, take some time to cool down, and then return. They need time to sort out what they are feeling.

Women, on the other hand, are the opposite. They feel more severely. It goes down to the core of their being. They want a solution right now. They do not want to wait. They want to deal with it. They want their partner to listen to them, even if it is just to vent. It does not necessarily mean a woman wants counsel; it just means that she wants her partner to hear what she is going through. A woman does not want her partner to ignore her, assume, or second-guess her. She wants him to know how she is feeling. Very often, in process of a fired-up conversation, a woman looks for answers to difficult questions and sometimes comes to understanding what it was all about and why she was thinking the way she was thinking.

## HOW A WOMAN TREATS A MAN

How a woman treats a man is dependent upon how she was raised. In Poland, young girls are trained to serve. We are raised to put a man's need before our own. We serve with no questions asked. Regardless if the man is educated or not, we are to serve. Women are not to seek social status, but to stay in the kitchen, tend to the children, clean house... that is just the way it is. With this type of upbringing, it does not matter if a woman is in pain or has a migraine headache. She must go on and complete her task either willingly or forcefully.

## A STRONG WOMAN

For me, I believe a real man is attracted to a woman who is strong and stands up for herself. A strong woman strives to create a positive environment for herself and her family. She is fun and outgoing. She believes in caring for others. She is not afraid to share her thoughts and ideas, regardless of the opposition. A strong woman speaks her heart and mind.

A strong woman challenges herself, is confident, and pushes herself to reach her greatest potential. She has a sense of humor, a willingness to learn, and asks questions. She puts one foot in front of the other, even when times are hard. She admits she does not have all the answers, but rather she continues to find knowledge and understanding. She has a hunger to learn, but can be a teacher when needed. A strong secure man is happy to listen to what she is really saying.

The bottom line is that, despite different ideas and what one believes, a couple can come to common ground. It is really okay to disagree; we all have a voice as long as we each converse respectfully without damaging each other's freedom.

## WHAT MEN NEED TO UNDERSTAND

When trying to communicate about complex issues like endometriosis, it is extremely vital for a man to be vigilant in his reaction. If he does not really understand the complexity of the disease, every word can make a remarkable difference.

Sometimes, there is nothing you can do or say that will make her feel better. Sometimes you will not have an answer, or an answer she wants to hear. The only thing you can do at this moment is show her that you care and that you are there for her. Embrace her with compassion and hold her close. (Physical touch is important.) Just to know that she has some support, that she is not alone, that she is with someone who cares about her may be all she needs to get her through that moment.

Nevertheless, even a strong woman can become weak and that is okay, and normal to feel this way - and to do so without regret. Today, I know that it is okay not to be strong sometimes. Forcing yourself to be strong, despite not feeling well, is honorable but not always the best path to take. It is okay not to deliver sometimes, and to not feel guilty. When you feel better you will catch up.

## KNOW YOURSELF

I encourage women to pursue and go after what they are good at. Try to find your element, and find out what you want in life and who you want to be. I think it is important to find out what you want from yourself, from others, and from life. Otherwise, you will remain incomplete. I also encourage you to educate yourself; it does not have to be formal because there are many ways to gain knowledge and experience. Looking for your element may take long and may take forever and both cases are totally ok. Some people find their element and stick to it for life, some of them have several of them and some people never find it. It is about the journey that makes it so enjoyable.

Knowing yourself is enlightening. There are women out there who do not know who they are and they do not realize their inner beauty. Maybe nobody told you that you are beautiful. Maybe no one told you that you are smart, or told you that you could do anything you want to do. Know that your strength comes from within. Your confidence in your strength comes from within. Nobody can give it to you, and no one should be able to take it away from you. I believe you can conquer anything. There are people who overcame the Holocaust, or a plane crash; in difficult times they found a way to survive.

## CREATE A VISION

Logic will take you from A to Z. Imagination will take you anywhere and everywhere you want to go. Imagine yourself being what you want to be, to be a creative vision of what you want to be as a woman. The Bible says in Genesis 2:18 that "it is not good for man to be alone, I'm going to make him a helper." Even God looked at a man as a perfect creation, yet he was incomplete without a woman. God gave him a gift in the shape of a woman. In a sense, we can say that the woman was the grand finale in creation. This tells me that women are overlooking their importance and significance in life. If God believes a woman is important, then you must believe that you are important. You are significant and have a purpose.

The greatest compliment that we can have is that we were created because the man was incomplete. That means we are needed. In the book of Proverbs, King Solomon describes a woman with great value.

> *A good one it is hard to find, and worth far more than diamonds.*
>
> *Her husband trusts her without reserve, and never has reason to regret it.*
>
> *Never spiteful, she treats him generously all her life long.*
>
> *She shops around for the best yarns and cotton, and enjoys knitting and sewing.*
>
> *She is like a trading ship that sails to the faraway places; it brings us back exotic surprises.*
>
> *She's up before dawn, preparing breakfast for her family and organizing her day.*

*She looks over a field and buys it, then, with money she puts it aside, and plants a garden.*

*First thing in the morning, she dresses for work, rolls up her sleeves, eager to get started. She senses the worth of her work, is in no hurry to call it quits for the day.*

*She skilled in the crafts of home and heard, diligent in homemaking.*
*She's quick to assist anyone in need, reaches out to help the poor.*

*She doesn't worry about her family when it snows; their winter clothes all mended ready-to-wear.*

*She makes her own clothing, and dresses in colorful linens and silks. Her husband is greatly respected when he deliberates with the city fathers.*

*She designs gowns and sells them, brings the sweaters she knits to the dress shops. Her clothes are well-made and elegant, and she always faces tomorrow with a smile.*

*When she speaks she has something worthwhile to say, and she always says it kindly. She keeps an eye on everyone in her household, and keeps them all busy and productive.*

*Children respect and bless her; her husband joins her with words of praise: "Many women have done wonderful things, but you've outclassed them all!"*

*Charm can mislead and beauty soon fades.*

*The woman to be admired and praised is a woman who lives in the fear of God.*

*Give her everything she deserves! Festoon her life with praises!*

*Proverbs 31:10-31 (MB)*

Even though King Solomon is praising the virtuous woman, we must understand that he was writing in a time when women were uneducated, living in a society and in a culture that required a woman to stay at home, tend to her children and that was the extent of her life. However, we must recognize that we live in a different culture and a different time. We must understand that good character and living life with integrity makes a great woman. In spite of your upbringing, or your lack of formal education, it should not stop you from believing that you can succeed at whatever you want to do in life.

Another example in the Bible is Esther who went before the King to save an entire nation. The king had such great power that a woman had no right to come before him without invitation. Yet she had great confidence in herself and her God that allowed her to go against accepted culture.

You were not created to be a doormat. You do not deserve to be disrespected or looked down upon by anybody. This does not give you a right to be mean or disrespectful, but it does mean that you have a right to be treated with honor. You need to have self-confidence and be open to talk about your strengths and weaknesses.

# CHAPTER 7 | Dealing with Pain

In this chapter, I would like to bring into perspective how endometriosis affects the daily routine and life of the woman. Endometriosis is a problem for more than 176 million women across the world. There are at least 8 million cases in the United States alone, according to the Endometriosis Research Center. It is one of the top three causes of infertility, it is the source of an estimated 80% of chronic pelvic pain, and accounts for more than half of the 600,000 hysterectomies performed annually. As I said before, a 2009 study calculated that costs of endometriosis care in the United States reached $69 billion in one year alone. [11]

---

[11] http://www.fitnessmagazine.com/health/body/pain- relief/endome triosis-symptoms/

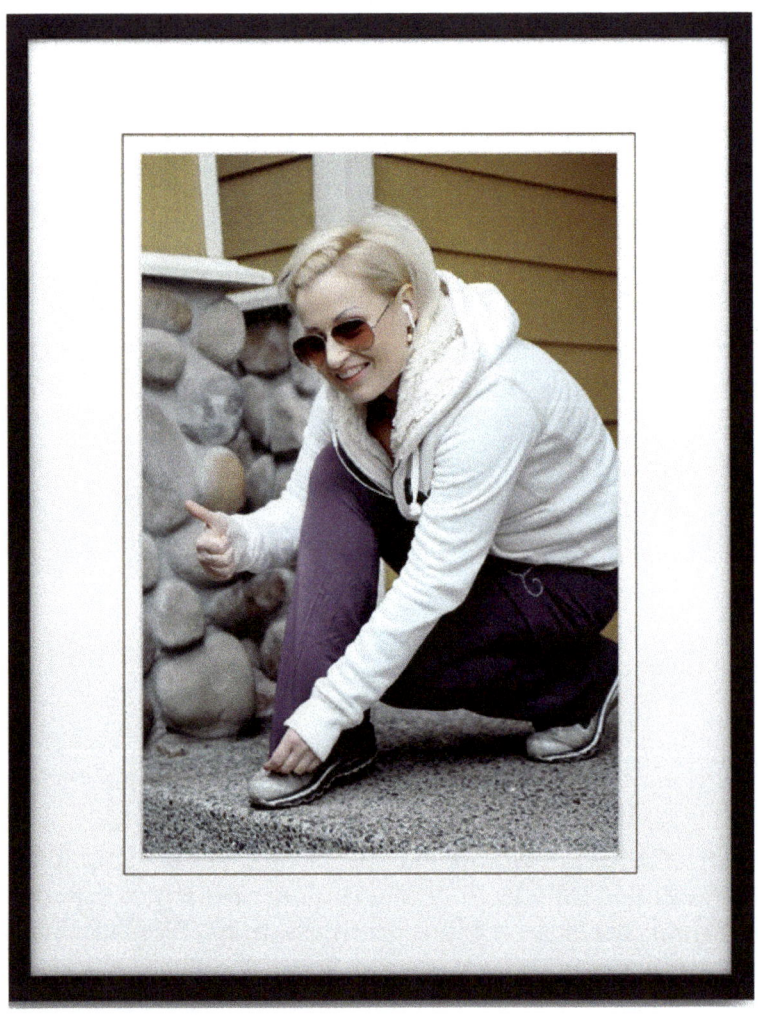

Because endometriosis pain most often occurs during ovulation, menstruation, urination, bowel movements, and sex, it has frequently dismissed or mistaken as a symptom of another health condition, which can lead to months or even years of misdiagnosis. This is especially true for younger women. "Studies indicate that up to 70% of teenagers with painful periods already have endometriosis," says Bruce Lessey, MD, PhD, a leading researcher of the condition and medical director of reproductive endocrinology and infertility at Greenville Hospital System University Medical Center in South Carolina. [12] Doctors regularly prescribe birth control pills as the first

---

[12] http://blog.ghs.org/2014/03/endometriosis/

line of defense against period pain, since moderating estrogen and progesterone levels has been shown to ease menstrual cramps. Lowering estrogen levels also eases endometriosis symptoms, however, so going on the pill may disguise the condition until a woman wants to start a family and discovers she can't conceive. [13]

## PAIN PAIN PAIN

The worst part of endometriosis is the continuous, constant chronic pain. It feels like a ripple of sudden, twinge-like pain. It can feel like the nerves in your abdomen have been signed with a hot iron. This pain stabs the area below the stomach and just above the groin area. To imagine the pain, think of the raw pain from a toothache. Now, imagine that feeling stuck perpetually somewhere deep inside your abdomen.

The pain doesn't have a pattern; it arrives and leaves as it wills. It can stay for hours, days, or weeks at a time. The pain is often accompanied by a tugging sensation, the felling that the area inside you is caught somehow, snagged on some unseen surface. Because you have no warning when it will hit, it can interrupt every aspect of your life.

Endometriosis affects the daily schedule and life of a woman. Typically, a woman is responsible for household chores educating herself and educating children. However, a woman who suffers from this disease will struggle to maintain a regular routine. It has been said that she will lose ten hours per week of productivity due to the disease. The physical challenges of losing that many hours will prevent her from doing consistent work in or out of the home. This creates internal and social problems, not only for the woman but also within her family.

---

[13] http://endosisters.weebly.com/about-endo.html

## LACK OF SELF-WORTH

The disease will create a lack of confidence and self-worth. It also affects a woman's educational choices, her future, and her level of success. Young girls are also struggling with their self-perception. The young girl is tired and weak all the time, and she can be appeared to be lazy or have no drive.

In my case, when it came to working, I was not only qualified but in many cases I was overqualified. But because of my illness, it affected me from always doing my best. At times, this could come across as if that I was not giving my full effort. However, I tried to do the I could all the time. I did not want to disappoint anyone so I tried to work harder to keep a good reputation. This is difficult for women because self-esteem and self-confidence are crucial to their inner strength.

After I graduated from high school and entered university, I had to miss numerous classes. I was very fortunate to be able to work this out with my teachers. I did not know yet what I was struggling with; all I knew was I was weak and losing focus, and was always tired. I loved studying and I knew that if I were in better heath I could be taking additional courses. Unfortunately, I could not do it at that time for unknown reasons. I was not a quitter, so I kept going but at the expense of my health. I was doing what I was taught to do: suck it up and keep going. I might also note that I was able to graduated top of my class in spite of my battle with what I would later learn was Endometriosis.

I can relate to many teenagers these days who also have limited physical abilities. Many girls cannot participate in sports because of the effects of endometriosis. Physical exercise is an important part of good health. However, the disease, in most cases, prevents them from having the strength for physical exercise.

If you are a wife or a mother, and your household is dependent upon two incomes in the household, the disease can become a great challenge. Without the proper support and understanding, you will not have the strength or feel confident in yourself.

## PSYCHOLOGICAL ASPECTS

The psychological aspects of this disease can result in isolation. Many times a woman will have to stay home from work or can end up in the hospital, causing her to feel guilty. She feels that she is disappointing others and letting them down. She is unable to participate in activities with her children. As a wife, she can feel guilty because she is not fulfilling her husband. This can cause anxiety and depression, and greatly affect her confidence.

From every angle, fear strikes: fear of disappointment, fear of being involved in a relationship, and fear of getting involved in intimate relationships. Fear of being excluded, because you cannot keep up or meet expectations. You may find yourself becoming angry–angry because you cannot keep up.

When it comes to psychological problems, this disease challenges your womanhood. Many of the emotional problems in your mind and the physical problems in your body can go undetected. Even though you might have a mental inclination that something is wrong, a medical approach will not consider it. The body and the mind are connected. The mental can cause physical problems and vice versa, so chronic pain affects us physically and psychologically.

When we think of pain, we must also think and understand how it affects us. The pain that we are dealing with causes anxiety. Pain affects our memory and our emotions. Remembering the pain can cause the pain to return. The mental anguish of anticipating the pain can bring unwanted distress. You think about how much it is going to hurt and then your brain begins to bring pain to your body. It is a vicious cycle, and the pain will bring stress and a perception of hopelessness.

Depression makes the pain even worse. Emotional issues are very important when we study pain. Physical pain alone can cause mental anguish. The mental pain brings physical pain.

Some people can deal easily with the pain and some people cannot. Some people can work with it and some cannot. We are all different and we are going to face pain individually. Our gender, our culture, and even our age will determine whether we can make sense out of anything. Pain can become an obsession. All of the physical and psychological aspects when dealing with pain will determine your well-being.

Dealing with pain for so many years, I could not find people who could understand, so I kept it to myself. For a good part of my life I had to cope with it myself. I did not seek help on how to deal with it mentally; everyone only wanted to treat me physically. Mental wellness was overlooked, and it caused me to suffer with great depression and phobia.

Do you recall earlier I said I had surgery? The doctor told me that I had a three month window to get pregnant. There was no discussion about what I was feeling, how to deal with relationships, or my emotions. I was just given the news that I had three months to get pregnant and after that, it would be impossible. How was I supposed to deal with that? I believe it is important for doctors not to overlook the mental and emotional side of this illness. I had limited hope of even carrying a baby full-term. Then there were questions about the baby's physical health. Would I survive? Would the baby survive? Would I be able to carry for nine months, or would it be a preemie? And if the infant was born premature, would it live a few days, and the die? The questions were overwhelming.

What a dilemma it is for a woman who wants a child! There is so much pressure to make a decision and choice.

This was a lot of for me to consider and contemplate, and I was getting very little support from others for my psychological wellness. In the beginning, I did not know the name of the disease, only the symptoms. The only thing I knew to do was to dig deep down inside and be determined to fight it. Most women are introverted and are tempted to crash, quit, and give up.

## PAIN AS MOTIVATION

My pain became my motivation. My pain became something positive. My pain led me to the light at the end of the tunnel. On the way to find information for this problem, I met other women who had the same symptoms. They inspired me to gain more knowledge and find a better way to cope. My desire was not only to discover more information, but also to discover the truth, and to help others with what I would find. It made me more open-minded and willing to face my struggles head on.

Moreover, I discovered my self-esteem. I began to reach out to other people. I felt needed again. I felt I could make a difference in other people's lives. I found out I was not alone. At some point, I even forgot about my pain when I saw other women who were suffering. Instead of just trying to cope, I felt their pain. I felt I could carry other people on my shoulders. This was a turning point for me; I was reminded that the reason I am on this earth is to help other people. I did not let my pain take me down. Instead, I learned from it.

I felt responsible for helping other people with their problems. I decided then to become an advocate for those who could not speak up. I wanted to motivate and inspire others. I gained experience and knowledge by working with many women who were suffering with this disease, as well as those who had suffered divorces, or were struggling with relationship issues. My goal was to help them see there is hope. I am very happy that I have learned how to cope and to live with pain.

Yes, I did everything I could, and tried everything possible when I started paying attention to how I truly felt, physically and emotionally. As long as I understood myself, I discovered I did not have to be alienated and forfeit my social life. I could cope with my pain, and I believe that my experience has enriched my life. I found the positive side of my pain. Everything that has had happened to me did so for a reason.

I believe it is important to see how extremely vital a woman is every part of society. Even though a woman thinks she limited, she is not.

I realize not everyone will have same approach and determination to overcome pain or to find the strength within. Making attempt however may take you places you may never think about but you will never know until you try. It feels good to look at yourself and be proud of what you have accomplished even it is not very significant in your opinion.

## NOT GOOD ENOUGH?

As a young girl, I was not strong physically. When I started having my menstrual cycle, my body changed rapidly and my mood swings increased. I withdrew from any activities and I could never keep up with my friends. I could not participate or keep up with any physical activities. On my better days, I could do aerobics and tennis. Despite my efforts, I was told I was not good enough. I was told I could not run fast or jump far. I could not put the basketball in the hoop when playing basketball. So I was always regarded as slow.

When I started my menstrual cycle at age 13, I needed more rest and more sleep. At that point, I had no clue why, but every ounce of strength was drained from me. No one had any idea that a disease was affecting my body.

When someone tells you are not good enough, you lose faith in yourself. You start believing their words. You believe that sports are not something for you. It is important to understand why someone is tired or feels weak. It is not necessarily because they are lazy but because something is wrong. That's why it is important to see signs and patterns. When I was dealing with a symptom, I had to take notice to understand what was happening.

I believe that if people would have understood me and knew what was wrong with me, I could have reached a greater potential. Even though I have achieved great goals, I could have done so much more. But many people put me down. Even though I have always been a social person, there were times where I did not want to be with other people.

## HOW YOUR BODY WORKS

In order to stay on track in your life, you must understand how endometriosis works, and how it will affect your body. You must understand that there are times that you will be productive and other times where you must slow down. It took me a few years to understand how my body functions. One week, I was doing great, and the next I would struggle. Nevertheless, I do not have to give up. I just simply have to recognize that I have good days and bad days. Keep in mind that a woman's body reacts to a cycle. Sometimes you will have downtime when your hormones begin to affect you negatively, and if you do not know the way endometriosis affects you, it will be hard for you to gain strength and to get back to where you need to be.

Young girls really always concern me. They are still learning what their body is all about. They are probably more shy, they do not know how to articulate their feelings and tend to go into "hermit zone."

So young girls can struggle and have difficulties that go undetected with this disease. They can fight this battle and struggle with this condition, and never have the proof of what is really happening.

Getting educated and knowing the symptoms will help young girls recognize the effects of the disease. Never diminish the potential in a young person! To chastise a young girl without proper diagnosis is a tragedy. Do not ignore symptoms. Be open-minded to what she is feeling and going through. Diagnosis for the disease can take up to ten years.

Knowing about endometriosis and observing girls is crucial. Coming across with initiative and calling it by name may solve a lot of future complications.

## NATURAL IS BEST

One of the factors when dealing with endometriosis is recognizing the source behind the disease. We must recognize what is environmental cannot be treated with conventional medicine. Conventional medicine attempts to treat the condition, symptoms, and the disease with unnatural medications. To treat this disease properly, it must be treated naturally. Each woman has a different hormonal level; therefore, one particular treatment cannot help every woman suffering with endometriosis. For instance, some women have excess bleeding and some do not. Some can exercise and some cannot. Scientific experiments with mice and rats have proven that certain foods can cause endometriosis.

I encourage women to understand that what they eat can affect their bodies. I say to every woman and to everybody not to eat manufactured foods. Things will not change overnight, but through having the right knowledge drastic changes will occur over time. When sharing with people who suffer with the disease, I educate them on the importance of eating right, even though some refuse to listen.

A doctor may not know how to treat you. As I said before: if the doctors do not know what causes the disease, how can they know how to treat it?
If this is the case, then how can anyone criticize you, if you choose to change your diet in an effort to help yourself? Listen to your body, get into your rhythm, and try to understand. Nobody will understand your body as well as you do. When it comes to food, your body will tell you what is good for you and what is not.

It was before in earlier chapters!!!!

---
### BE CONSCIOUS
---

It is very important to listen to your body and to pay attention to what it is telling you. Perhaps you are a person who is sensitive to drugs and medicines. Maybe certain foods cause your stomach to be upset. It is so important to listen to even the smallest clue, if you truly want to be able to track the effects of endometriosis on your body, soul, and mind.

For instance, if you are open to it, consider acupuncture. Chronic pain, hormonal imbalances, and digestive problems often respond well to alternative treatments.

I know you want to take care of your body, and exercise is a good thing. However, too much exercise might having adverse effects on you. As well, exercising during the week prior to your menstrual cycle can be very beneficial because sweating cleanses the lymph nodes, and endometriosis is often affected by toxicity.So you have to monitor yourself. Remember, slow and steady wins the race.

Do not be afraid to seek out a nutritionist, a herbalist, or other natural naturalists. Here are a few more dietary changes to consider:

- Honey is actually an anti-inflammatory sweetener.
- Avoid homogenized milk; it is one of the most inflammatory food items in grocery stores today.
- Stay clear of all soy products. Soy contains phytoestrogens, which are compounds that mimic estrogen in the body. They can cause major hormone instability, which will worsen the endometriosis.
- Avoid processed foods because almost all of them contain chemical additives will inflame your endometriosis.
- Drink only pure spring water to avoid chorine found in municipal drinking water.

Do not neglect your psychological makeup. Perhaps a life coach or a good counselor can help you. Be open to address issues such as:

- Feeling like a helpless victim who lacks control over her life.
- Feeling "less than" a woman.
- Strained relationships, including family, spousal, coworkers, and doctor-patient.
- Being treated in a dismissive and disrespectful ways.
- Not being believed.
- Missing out on activities.

Do not give up! My life has become extraordinary and I believe that yours can too. I am no longer on hormone therapy. I am no longer on pain medicine. I am only taking some medicine for my liver that has been damaged over time. I worked on it for five long years, consistently, patiently through tears and doubts and trials. I had moments when I didn't know if what I was doing was really helping. I was confused numerous times, I didn't know if I was really getting better or it was just my wishful thinking. It was really the longest trip I have ever taken. Making a day it was a project, following all the riles and doing all the cleanses, juices and taking natural remedies. Sometimes I felt like I am 100 years old, thinking only how I feel and what I need to take. I developed fear of taking and swallowing pills, it was my phobia. It worked and I am a living example.

I am hoping for a day when doctors will find a happy medium. I believe that endometriosis can be treated with certain medications, while in other cases surgery may be needed. My point is you need to take the time to find out what you need to do, what is best for your body.

I combined traditional/alternative medicine with conventional. I think these two can work together. I am not saying to ignore your doctor's advice; he or she may show you some things that may work for you. I am saying: take it all, try it all using your common sense and listening to your inner voice, you will make the right decision.

## BE YOUR OWN MASTER

You cannot find an instant remedy. There is no such thing. But you can become your very own master. Share your pain until you no longer have it. Find what works for you... and you will once again begin to be the person you were meant to be. Be curious, always.

# CHAPTER 8
## Dealing with Pain

Few subjects matter more to people than health. Everyone wants to be healthy. However, good health can be elusive, as can be seen by the numbers of people who have health problems and complaints. It seems that more people are sick today than ever before.

Illness dramatically challenges marriages. When one mate becomes chronically ill, while the other remains healthy, complications can multiply quickly and if not addressed, it can spin things out of control.

Sadly, too many marriages have not survived the strain caused by a chronic disease such as endometriosis. Yet, this does not mean that a marriage is doomed to failure. The illness is not at fault; it is how the couple copes with it and if they choose to work together as a team that matters.

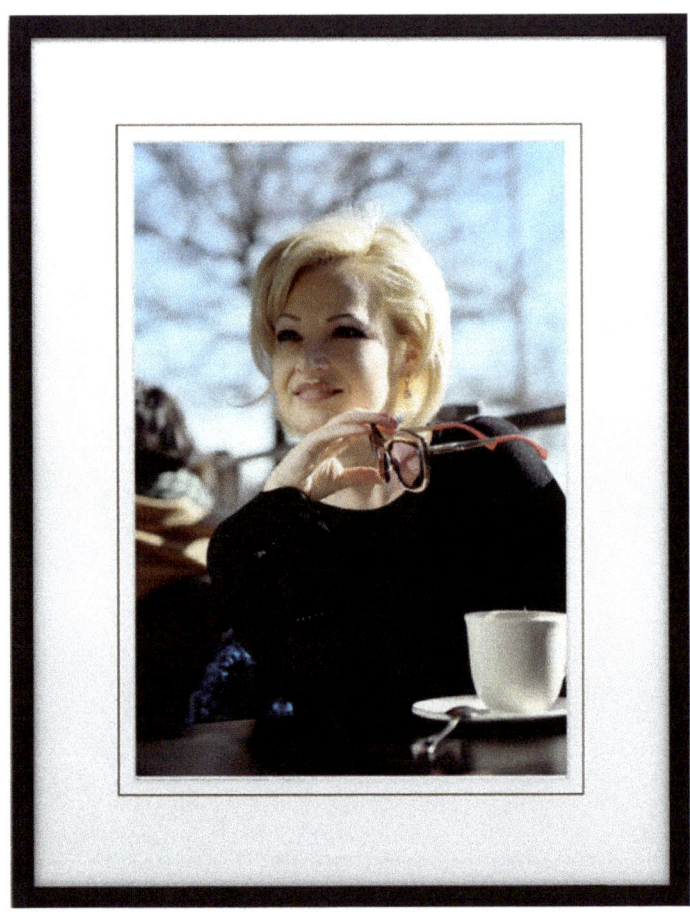

## RELATIONSHIPS AND ENDOMETRIOSIS

In this chapter, I would like to talk about the relationships between men and women in the context of dealing with endometriosis.

It is important for both parties to work together. Education is key. Nelson Mandela said, "No country can really develop unless its citizens are educated." He also said, "Education is the most powerful weapon which you can use to change the world." [14] I would add, "A lack of knowledge is a choice."

---

[14] http://thoughtjoy.com/nelson-mandela 41

Having a disease and chronic pain can cause incredible amounts of stress and strain on a relationship. However, it can also be an opportunity for a couple to grow in their relationship. When an illness occurs, people tend to put more focus upon the ill person. That is because a sickness weakens the person, and they struggle to cope with their pain. For example, someone who is always dependent upon others may become increasingly unable to function alone, while someone who is more independent may become increasingly isolated.

This has a detrimental effect upon relationships. Relationships that are already weak are likely to suffer the most. When partners lack communication skills, or do not try to talk, they are the ones most likely to accuse and to be slow to forgive. When fighting this disease, it can be a crippling blow to the relationship.

## WHY DOES HE DO THAT?

Many women who have endometriosis do not understand why their partner acts the way he does. They ask themselves, "Why does he not want to be involved with my situation? Why does he not believe I am in chronic pain? Why is he so quiet when I am hurting? Why is he more concerned when he will have sex? How can I meet his physical needs when sexual activity is so painful? Why will he not get involved?"

These questions imply that your partner understands your pain and disease, when he does not. First, for a man, the entire menstrual cycle is a foreign experience. Now, add the disease and it is even more confusing. For example, a common question a man asks is, "If the problem is with her reproductive organs, why does my partner blame her fatigue on endometriosis?" If the man refuses to be educated, he will not understand what his partner is going through. The man and the woman must become co-students or the relationship will likely dissolve.

I encourage you to talk more about the relationship, and talk less about the illness. Worry less, show more consideration for each other, and have a mutual interest outside the illness. Have more social contact, have mutual goals or a hobby; anything that causes you to work together. Begin there first, and work together the same way when it comes to tackling this disease.

## MEN, BECOME EDUCATED ON ENDO

I encourage men to get familiar with endometriosis. You will probably find out how little you have known until now, or you may even realize you really do not known nothing it at all. Or perhaps, you will learn from other women and their experiences. Hearing it from a different person can bring new understanding to your situation. You might discover that others facing the same disease are succeeding. Therefore, you can too.

I can tell you that each time I talk to a man about endometriosis and I make it more approachable, meaning I translate it to his language, I always hear, "Wow this is sad. This is horrible. I did not know it was this serious!"

Since we are talking about something invisible, it may be very hard to describe, imagine, and feel. However, when you tell a man to imagine it on his own body, it may be more engaging.

Recently, I saw a document that describes how a man would feel if he was a woman suffering pain during child delivery. The men were connected to wires that were sending sharp pain, creating symptoms as if they were in labor. After this very short experience, which only lasted a fraction of the normal time it takes to deliver a baby, each man decided he would not like to give birth. They had a greater respect for women and, no doubt, became more sympathetic for the female process of childbearing.

Whenever your partner is suffering, it is necessary to see, hear, and better understand what she is going through. In the matter of endometriosis, it gets a little tricky, because many women do not know what they are dealing with themselves. Since the diagnosis takes so long, she just cannot figure out what is happening to her, let alone name the condition. The only way she can articulate her feelings is to express them using very common words, such as pain, a headache, a migraine, or excessive tiredness. Why would anyone assign these symptoms, apparently so common to any particular disease?

Men tend to want to fix things because that is their nature - they are fixers. Like working on an automobile, or remodeling the garage into a man cave, they like to fix stuff and solve problems. They like to suggest things, like an expert telling you what is wrong and how to fix it. However, a man cannot find an "instant fix" for this disease. And he can make matters worse by approaching it without having enough knowledge.

## OPEN CONVERSATION

Unfortunately, we have a clash going on between men and the women. Women, we are different. We like to talk about things. We are open, and want to discuss things without hesitation. Women are heart-led and emotionally centered. We like to get things off our chest. Men do not normally want to talk about things. They hold their feelings inside and talk less than a woman. Ask a women how her day went, and she will give her man a play-by-play, moment-by-moment description of each event and every comment relative to the daily events. Ask a man how his day went and he will answer the woman in one word, "Fine." Talking about it is the first step. But what do you do when you do not know?

Now when we consider a woman with endometriosis, we really do not see what is wrong. She does not look like she is sick or suffering. She is beautiful. She is inspiring. She looks great. Therefore, it is so easy to deny the existence of the disease.

Open conversation between men and women is vital. We must understand that sometimes we women need to be left alone after having a bad day. Sometimes we need our space to get our peace of mind. Not because we do not want to be with a man, but because when we feel bad, we do not feel good about ourselves. We want to isolate ourselves. This is how women react to it. Women are very critical of their appearance. When we do not feel good, we automatically think we do not look good, and even if we may be perceived completely differently, it is very hard to convince us otherwise.

## A CAUTIONARY TALE

Let me tell you again about Dagny, my English teacher when I was a young girl. She was a wonderful and a beautiful woman. She was always healthy, until she got older and she started limping. Because she was so well known as a beautiful actress, when her limp became very noticeable, she did not want people to see her like that, so she spent all her time at home. How sad.

There were times when I wanted to defend her. I wanted to protect her, which was a natural thing for me to do. To me, she was beautiful despite of her limping or age because I loved her. Yet she saw herself quite differently than I did.

## WHAT A WOMAN NEEDS

Because women suffer, at times, with identity crisis or a low self-image, it is even more important for a man to recognize what she is going through emotionally. I think that a man needs to exercise more compassion and become more cordial. It is very important for him not to assume anything. Assumptions are the termites of relationships. We can assume something that is not right. We need to talk openly. We need to make time for conversation. We need to listen, not only hear things.

Because men are more logical, they are unlikely to participate with doctor visits. However, it is always better for the couple to hear what the doctors have to say together, and to hear the opinion of someone respected on health matters. It is more likely for your partner to acknowledge your health condition, and more likely to change his attitude towards you and your behavior when he hears it from a professional.

Sometimes, until we hear about something we will not touch it. We just cannot get it, but this is part of human nature. That would be a pity if someone would insist on denying the importance of a matter, especially in this case, when studies show this disease can be deadly if not treated correctly.

Going to the doctor with your partner will make the disease impossible to deny. Both of you will better understand that this is not just something in her head. Many women are accused of this. They are accused of making it up or trying to get sympathy.

I deeply believe this is a major reason why woman with endometriosis are getting depressed. They scream to be noticed, understood, and acknowledged. They are facing so much denial and ignorance from loved once and professionals, the rejection is overwhelming. It takes lots of time and energy to convince so many people around us we are really having a problem. Hopefully, understanding the differences in our natures can give us a better clue as how to talk, listen, and understand each other.

## HOW MEN ARE MADE

Women, on the other hand, should understand the difference in how men are created. Women cannot expect their partner to know what she thinks or feels. Endometriosis cannot be seen or touched readily. Therefore, a man cannot read your mind. You must tell him how and where you hurt. With men, some may be very insensitive to pain, or have never had an experience where pain immobilized them. They do not understand or sympathize naturally with the intense pain that endometriosis can bring. You cannot expect your partner to guess how you feel. Remember, women say one thing, mean another, and men hear something totally different. Your partner should not have to guess what you are trying to say.

For example, I have a friend whose husband asked her what she wanted for her birthday. She said, "Oh, you really don't need to get me anything." She told him, "Don't worry about it; just bring yourself." What she really meant was she was hoping he would be creative enough to come up with something she would not have to spell out so obviously.

So he took it as she said, literally. When the birthday party came, many people showed up and he was the only one without a present, because he took her literally. But really what she meant was not that she was happy for him not to buy her something; it was a way of saying that she was grateful for whatever he would get her.

## COMMUNICATION IS THE KEY

Communication is the key. When you are dealing with your partner, the more that you share with him, the easier it is for him to understand this disease.

Do not isolate. It is important to open up because you need each other. Your partner needs to understand that the pain is so unbearable that you want to be alone. But it is also the most important time to have somebody with you.

Men, understand that we want to be alone but we do not want to feel alone; that may sound very difficult for you to understand. It is a very misunderstood topic. The condition of endometriosis can cause the relationship and the partnership to fall apart, if you are not careful. Women, when discussing your pain, be specific. Show your partner where you hurt. Tell your partner what you really feel. Ask for help. You might be surprised at what your partner has noticed and the comfort he can provide.

Involve your partner with the process when selecting a physician. Discuss it together. Do your research before choosing a doctor. You *want* a doctor who will educate you and your partner about endometriosis. Find someone who will take the time to explain what is going on inside your body. But, realize that some doctors may be intimidated, or feel uncomfortable having your partner with you. If that were the case, I suggest looking for another doctor.

It is important to have a doctor who understands vulnerable patients and who knows how to share the information, as well as how to minimize mental and psychological damage.

After my surgery, I was told I had only three months to get pregnant! I was not asked if I had a partner or if I was in a relationship. What was it supposed to mean to me then? Was I supposed to go on a street and find anyone just to make sure I would be a fulfilled woman who delivered a child to this world?

I was told if I do not did not pregnant, then I would have to undergo another surgery before getting pregnant or I would have to take hormones. I was mature enough and educated enough not to take it to the extreme. Nevertheless, I could only imagine how a woman might feel if she was struggling to become pregnant.

## EDUCATION IS ESSENTIAL

Communicate with your partner about the changes in your body, the mood swings, and the emotional high and lows. If you feel your partner is not sympathetic to your pain, be cautious not to get angry or say it in a way that puts him on the defense. Instead, get pamphlets, find articles and websites that explain the disease and read them together.

For men, one of the biggest struggles will be intercourse, and the lack of it. It is extremely rare for any man to experience anything that interferes with his sex drive. Even more so, it is uncommon for sexual intercourse to cause pain with a man. He does not understand that endometriosis can suppress libido. This will make it difficult for a man to understand how the disease can interfere with a woman's sex drive.

Many times, a woman will not want to disappoint her partner, so she will endure the pain that comes with intercourse and not say anything. If this is the case, it becomes difficult to be enthusiastic or responsive to romantic endeavors. A lack of interest can cause your partner to think that you do not love him. He may assume that he have failed to satisfy you, or that you are angry with him.

If this area is not addressed, the relationship is sure to fall apart. Men and women approach sexuality differently, and they may not understand the importance of caressing, cuddling or touching. Do not let painful intercourse keep you from other forms of sexual expression. Let your partner know what you need and be creative to meet his. The answer is not abstinence, but options. Spend time developing a plan that will assist you with enjoying physical intimacy. Your partner cannot misread you in this area, or it will created bigger problems, such as an affair, separation or divorce.

Women, you do not need to feel isolated. Getting sick is a family affair. When you are dealing with any health condition, it is important that you gain support from your partner, your children or your parents. You might not be able to perform the way you should without support. It is important that everyone contribute to the happiness of the one who is suffering. Otherwise, the family will fall apart.

Men, it is important that you make your woman feel confident and that she is important. It is something very uncomfortable for a woman to discuss. We cannot avoid the problem. It is not like just having a cup of coffee, sitting down, and talking about it. It is important to open up and get to know each other. Because there is so little information about endometriosis, it is difficult to talk about your feelings.

## ENDOMETRIOSIS AND SEX

Endometriosis affects a woman psychologically and mentally. So when it comes to having intercourse, she may suffer acute pain. People will do almost anything to avoid pain. So if she denies her man sexual intercourse, he often gets confused and discouraged. A man and woman must come together and give 100% to get through this. Learning about this disease will open up ways for you to try to handle the situation.

It is very important for a man to show his woman that he cares, rather than showing frustration or irritation. Ask yourself, "Why is my partner so quiet when I am hurting?" Men have been trained since childhood to provide and protect his mate. When a man watches his partner endure chronic pain that he can do nothing about, it threatens his manhood. He feels helpless to save her from something that is ruining the quality of her life.

Sometimes, a man withdraws because he feels that there is no way to fight the enemy, and so he throw up his hands, defeated, wondering what to do. It is difficult to comfort someone when you feel that you have let them down. Therefore, the result may be silence. If this happens, let him know that you do not expect him to fix the problem. Remind him that it is no one's fault that you have endometriosis. Instead, tell your partner how much his closeness means to you. Just knowing that you want comfort will ease his worry and makes him feel he can do something. Stress the fact that he has not let you down.

Women, if you do not discuss your illness, your man may become pushy. It will not be easy but you must work through it. You relationship is too important to let it go by.

Men must understand that the pain is not always physical; it is also mental. Trust is very important. Talking about sexuality and what you enjoy is not easy, but when you can let go of your feelings and can open up, you will find success.
Self-esteem is important with men, and if you diminish his perception of you, he will feel rejected.

## ARTICULATE YOUR FEELINGS

In Emotional Intelligence by Daniel Goleman, the author discusses how to articulate your feelings. Too many times, conversations are empty. Even though all the words seem perfect, nothing is really being said. It does not matter if you take your woman out for dinner or buy her flowers, if you do not understand and communicate about this, nothing you do will help.

We as women need to let men approach us. We need to let them do so because sometimes the ways in which we communicate, we can hurt them mentally. We need to be very cautious and try to prevent it from happening. If you feel bad just say, "If I behave or say something ugly, please don't take it too personally. I am having a very bad day." Or, "I'm struggling with my feelings today, so if I say something too harsh, please don't let hurt you." Many times, I did not know that I was even feeling or acting that way.

In order for the relationship to work, the two of you must become best friends. A friend is not someone who was there just when you are happy but when you cry. Someone you can call when you are down. My mom always used to tell me it is more important to go to the funeral home, then to a party house. I never did understand that as a child. Now I understand it because there is nothing more important than to be there when someone really needs you. There is nothing worse than to be sick and have nobody there.

Nothing is worse than to be lonely when you are going through problems or illness. This is why I want to emphasize the closeness of the relationship. Physical touch is important. Isolating yourself and withdrawing does not help. This can be easy when you are in a relationship where you each know the other and your emotional needs.

Men, eye contact is important. It is an emotional way to show that you care and are concerned. It is important to talk about things. Ask her what she wants. During hurtful times sometimes, she might want to be alone and other times she may want comfort.

## FIVE LOVE LANGUAGES

I recommend the book The Five Love Languages by Gary Chapman. When I read this book, I learned so much about love. The book talks about different ways of feelings and emotions and how people show love in different ways. Some men, when trying to show their women that they love her, will wash her car. But for some women, this would not matter; they may feel that spending time together is the best way to show love. The book will help couples find their "love language" as well as their partner's.

## JUST LET GO

As funny as it sounds, women are crazy. Yes, I said it we are crazy. Men and women do not think the same. Ladies, you cannot expect men to understand you when you cannot understand yourself. They need to hear things as they are, not as we want them to be. We can save ourselves so much aggravation when we approach men differently. Your man will always ignore you if you leave it up to him to guess what you are thinking.

I think three words would best conclude it: "Just let go!" I sometimes look back and recall certain situations and I must admit that I must have driven a particular man insane! I laugh because it was really my fault, but I wanted to make point of it with him, or maybe I did not want to do anything I was just stubborn.

When a woman gets to know one man well, she can say she knows most men. However, if a man gets were to get to know every woman, he cannot tell if he knows even one of them.

Men, when you ask a woman if it is okay to do something and they say, "Do whatever you want" that usually means they do not want you to do it. This is an example of not understanding what we mean when we say something.

It is very hard for men to understand a woman, because we do not even understand ourselves. Sometimes we want this and then later we don't want it anymore. Our feelings are under hormonal construction. So sometimes, we must be asked what we mean by how we act.

Do not try to understand a woman. Love her and respect her. Do not take everything so personally. When woman is going through menopause or a menstrual cycle, it affects her emotions, her mood, and her thinking. The change of moods and emotions are hard to read.

We must learn to laugh and not take everything so serious. It is hard to deal with this disease. But it is not the end of the world. I really believe that if you put your mind to it you can make a difference. Even though you deal with pain, what are you willing to contribute to your life? You have to have a positive attitude.

You cannot allow anything, anyone, or any condition to control your life. I believe that if you have a partner who knows what you are dealing with, the relationship has a chance to last. Men and women you must stick together.

# CHAPTER 9
# Secret Suffering

It is an old myth that young girls do not get endometriosis. Far too many doctors still believe that endometriosis is rare in teenagers and young women. Consequently, they do not consider a diagnosis when teenagers and young women complain of symptoms like period pain, pelvic pain, and painful intercourse.

In fact, some research indicates that up to two thirds of women with endometriosis have symptoms before they are 20 years old. This means that symptoms in adolescent girls need to be taken seriously, while still recognizing that not all menstrual pain symptoms are necessarily due to the disease.

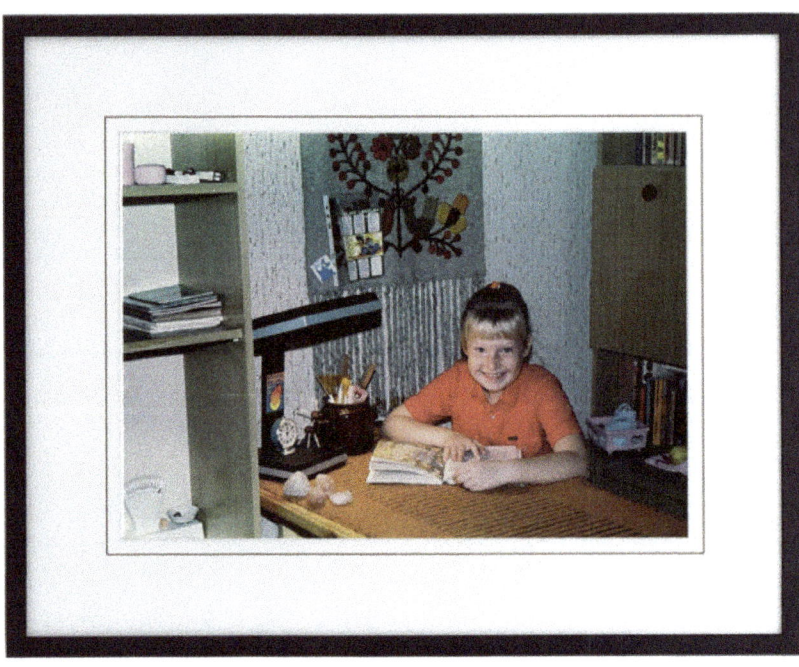

Unfortunately, this belief is a carry-over from earlier times. Before the introduction of laparoscopy in the 1970s, endometriosis could only be diagnosed with a major surgery involving a roughly four to five inch incision into the abdomen. The risks and costs of such surgery meant it was usually done only as a last resort in women with the most severe symptoms who were past childbearing age. Because only women in their 30s or 40s were operated on, the disease was only found in women of that age. Subsequently "the fact" arose that endometriosis was a disease of women in their 30s and 40s.

### LAPAROSCOPY CHANGED DIAGNOSIS

It was only with the introduction in the 1970s and 80s of laparoscopy to investigate women with infertility problems that gynecologists began diagnosing the disease in women in their late 20s and early 30s. Thus, they revised the typical age range for endometriosis down to this age group. Again, they did not consider that they might be "finding" it because they were "looking" for it. [15]

---

[15] http://endometriosis.org/resources/articles/myths/

The realization that endometriosis could be found in teenagers and young women came about because of research by the national endometriosis support groups in the mid-1980s, which caught the attention of some eminent gynecologists in the 1990s. Dr. Marc Laufer of the Children's Hospital Boston conducted studies of teenagers with chronic pelvic pain. One of his studies showed that adolescents, whose chronic pelvic pain was not alleviated by an oral contraceptive pill and a non-steroidal anti-inflammatory drug like Ponstan, had a high prevalence of endometriosis - as high as 70%. [15]

Most recently, the Global Study of Women's Health, conducted in sixteen centers in ten countries, showed that two thirds of women sought help for their symptoms before the age of 30, many experiencing symptoms from the start of their first period.

Teenagers and young women in their early 20s are not too young to have endometriosis. In fact, most women experience symptoms during adolescence, but unfortunately are not diagnosed and treated until they are in their 20s or 30s.

If you are a teenager, and you have menstrual pain to the extent that it keeps you away from school, or it prevents you from participating in day-to-day activities, then you should discuss your symptoms with your doctor.

## CONSULTING THE DOCTOR

In order to prepare for a first consultation with your doctor, you may want to print off a paper with your symptoms, your questions, and any other things you want to be sure to remember to talk about. When you are researching about endometriosis, you can find all lists of symptoms, which are good to have on you to help you remember. Sometimes when a young girl/ teenager visits a gynecologist, she

---

[16] http://www.livingwithendometriosis.org/myths/
[17] www.womenshealth.gov/publications/our-publications/fact-sheet/infertility.html

may not feel yet very comfortable talking about her symptoms. Having a paper with the symptoms you are experiencing may help you keep it all together. This can act as an aid in your discussions.

It will help you to think about your symptoms, when they occur, and how often. Make sure that you mention everything you want to talk about during the consultation with your physician. It can be hard to remember everything you wish to discuss without writing it down ahead of time, and a list may aid you. It may also help your physician to understand your particular situation better.

Please remember doctors see many patients every day. They really want to bring you relief. Having you over and over again in his office with the same symptoms is must be very disturbing for both parties. Proper articulation and even suggestion maybe extremely helpful. Misdiagnosing endometriosis is extremely easy.

## TWO EARS ARE BETTER THAN ONE

For your first consultation, you may also want to bring one of your parents or a good friend, with you: two sets of ears are better than one, and your companion can help you remember all the information the physician may give you about your treatment options.

Do not be afraid of asking questions. The physician is there to help you. If there is something you do not understand, or something you feel you need to know more about, then ask.

## TREATMENT OPTIONS

The treatment options do not vary that much, whether you are a teenager or a woman in her 20s, 30s, or 40s. (See Appendix I for a brief discussion of some of the treatments offered by conventional medicine. See Appendix II for an overview of the some of the alternative treatments.)

As with any treatment, the key component is learning what is appropriate for your symptoms, and being comfortable with the therapy you are undergoing. You are the one to decide to what extent you are able and willing to deal with any side effects of any treatment! You need to discuss these options carefully with your physician, so that together you can find the best and most effective treatment for your specific symptoms. Do not rush these decisions. Again, never be afraid to ask questions if there is something, you are not sure about.

# CHAPTER 10 | Deciding on Treatment

It is an old myth that young girls do not get endometriosis. Far too many doctors still believe that endometriosis is rare in teenagers and young women. Consequently, they do not consider a diagnosis when teenagers and young women complain of symptoms like period pain, pelvic pain, and painful intercourse.

In fact, some research indicates that up to two thirds of women with endometriosis have symptoms before they are 20 years old. This means that symptoms in adolescent girls need to be taken seriously, while still recognizing that not all menstrual pain symptoms are necessarily due to the disease.

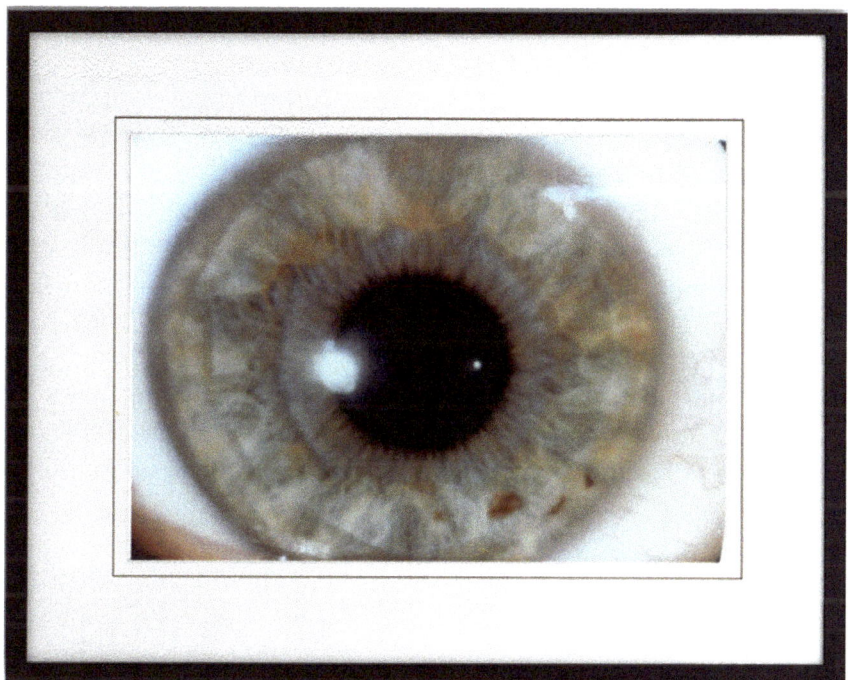

The ability to make the right decision is extremely vital, especially in health matters. It can be also very stressful. In that particular matter, I believe that you should make any final decisions, as long as you are mentally capable.

As much as I believe what doctors say, I've learned one very important thing: I am the person who will deal with the results. Hence, I should be the person to decide which path of treatment I will take. I am always open to hear what a particular doctor has to say and recommend, but I follow up on their advice with my own research and study.

This chapter is not to judge or criticize anyone in the medical field or any medication that is prescribed. Each person must judge and follow their own path in battling endometriosis.

## CONVENTIONAL VS. ALTERNATIVE MEDICINE

An article in *The Journal of the American Medical Association* says, "Opening a professional dialogue between physicians and practitioners of alternative medicine is crucial to better health care for those patients who choose alternative therapies." The article goes on to say "This need [of dialogue] can be expected to grow with use of alternative therapies, particularly as health insurance plans include such therapies in the benefits they offer."

More and more patients are employing alternative therapies while availing themselves of other conventional forms of treatment. Yet, some fail to keep their medical doctor informed of what they are doing.

Therefore, Tufts University Health Nutrition Letter of April 2000 urged, "You should act in your best interest by working with your doctor rather than privately." The letter added, "Whether he or she approves of your approach, you still stand to gain by sharing the information."

This was said because of possible health risks when certain herbs are combined with conventional therapies. Recognizing that some of their patients are choosing alternative therapies, many health professionals strive not to allow their own opinions about health care to prevent them from working along with alternative therapists for the benefit of the patient.

Such it was in my case. While searching for help, answers and doctors, I came across almost anything and anyone who appeared to me as a professional. From conventional to alternative medicine, I feel I have covered it all.

I used conventional medicine for all sorts of tests and for my surgery after which I felt 100% better for some period of time. Then, I turned to alternative ways of healing. I exposed myself to almost anything. I have to admit, It looked very weird at times. Everything helped to some degree; therefore, I achieved the most favorable results.

---

[10] November 11, 1998

Our modern world has forced us to grow accustomed to taking drugs for every common aliment. However, we have not been educated to understand that we cannot fool our bodies by man-made preparations with frequently dangerous side effects. We can only fool our mindsets.

## A NEW THERAPY

In For Your Eyes Only, Frank Navati, BSC N.D. writes, "Surprisingly, we already have at our disposal the most naturally sophisticated tool for diagnosing, not only a disease, but most importantly, the causes of the disease. It is something that most of us possess - our eyes. Yes, these magnificent organs allow us to view the world around us, and act as a map to every organ, gland, and system in your body."

After reading his book I decided to visit an iridologist. I really had no clue what to expect, but I went with my gut feeling and I am glad I did. I found out about this intriguing world and a fascinating branch of alternative medicine. I learned that eyes are not only the windows to our souls; they are also hidden maps to our bodies. As Navarti says, "Iris diagnosis is the only real method that at glance can provide a wonderful true picture of a patient's entire health status."

Imagine this: I am sitting in a small room, not even remotely resembling a doctor's office. I see a microscope, quite old I must say, nothing fancy. If I acted on my initial judgment, I probably would have left. However, the lady who worked with me had a way about her, which convinced me to just give it a try. I did not tell her, prior to my visit, what I was struggling with. She took a picture of my iris and went over it with me. This was amazing experience. Not only did she tell me what I struggle with, she told me what I struggled with in my childhood. She told me things I did not remember at first; things that really happened.

For the first time, I was recommended supplements that helped me with my chronic fatigue. I actually started feeling better and stronger almost immediately. I felt as if I was taking off my mask, and was ready to spread my wings again.

"I believe this iris diagnosis is the most precise form of diagnosis that exists, and as more research is made in it, it may become the method of choice of diagnosis in the future." Navarti says.

This visit opened me the world of alternative medicine to me. Getting my energy back didn't completely satisfy me, but it was a milestone. I was still struggling with pain and all other endometriosis symptoms, so I did not stop searching.

## TRADITIONAL CHINESE MEDICINE

In my workplace, we continually discussed healthy living, eating, and all the alternatives. A friend of mine mentioned a Chinese doctor she knew. I had not tried this avenue as of yet so I decided to pay him a visit. What would I lose? $100 compared to the $1,000s I had already spent was worth it to me. At his office, I was surprised by the number of people in the waiting room. That was a good sign. Although the scent in the room was not exactly fragrant, I assumed it have must emanated from the herbs.

## MY MASTER GUO

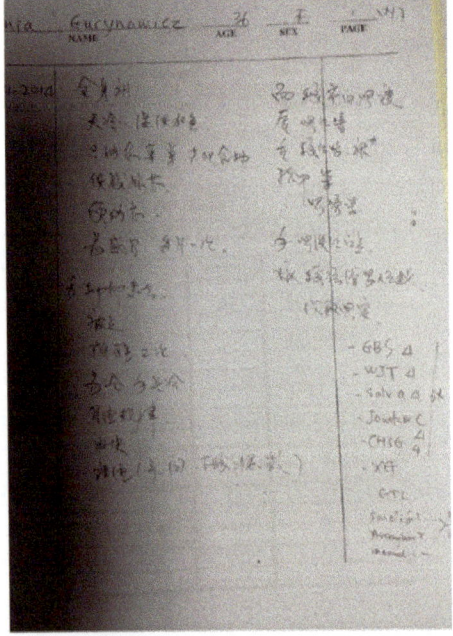

An older man opened the door, and struggled to call my name properly. I got up and just introduced myself with my first name "Ania." We shook hands and went to his room.

The room only contained his desk, his chair, and couple of chairs for his patients. There were no posters on the walls showing human anatomy; there were no any devices, just a very old phone.

He looked at my face and he

said, "Pale, very pale." Then he asked me to give him my hand so he could check my pulse. While he doing so, he was also taking notes in Chinese! It was pretty amusing to me. He looked at my tongue and that was it. He knew everything. My visit lasted exactly ten minutes. He said, "Severe, your pain is severe, but it shouldn't be like this, I will help you."

I was speechless, and to be honest, I was so surprised by the entire procedure that I did not know what to ask about. I did not have any questions. Because of his age, I might have taken his diagnosis for granted. Nevertheless, the whole procedure was very mysterious.

> He sent me to the front desk where I was to pick up my natural remedies. I decided to try his diagnosis, and bought all I needed to start this "experiment." I was amazed! For the first time after years of trying to break free from all the pain and all endometriosis syndromes, I knew this was working.
>
> I became curious who this man was, and how did he know so quickly how to help me. This is what I found out.
>
> Zhengang Guo, our master herbalist and acupuncturist, established Life Rising in 1985 after dual life-long pursuits in both (TCM) and Western medicine. His background in TCM began as a teenager in his native village of Lanzhou when his father, Xiang-Li Guo, personally taught his children the fundamentals of TCM, a field that began over two thousand years ago.
>
> With his extensive knowledge of TCM, Guo attended the Lanzhou Medical College to train as a Western surgeon and oncologist. After graduating, he practiced throughout northwest China for 17 years. Ultimately, Guo envisioned the potential of integrating the best of Western medicine with TCM, thus, he immigrated to the United States in 1981 on a fellowship with the M.D. Anderson Tumor Hospital in Houston, Texas.
>
> Later, he moved to Chicago where he continued his research at the University of Illinois and began the first Chinese herbal

medicine class ever taught in the Windy City. Because Guo made inroads at that time, anyone with the desire to become a TCM practitioner or an acupuncturist in Chicago now has more opportunity. Furthermore, The College of Medicine at The University of Illinois is now known for its legitimizing research in alternative medicine therapies.

While living in the US, Guo realized that the factors affecting his Western patients varied greatly from his patients in China. One of his first challenges was to adapt the traditional formulas to his new patients' needs. Next, Guo faced the problem of the West's unfamiliarity with TCM's principles and philosophy as well as the tastes, smells, and lengthy preparation times for its herbal medicines. Master Herbalist Guo has made remarkable developments to improve TCM's tastes and smells. Thanks to his extensive research, the preparation of herbs for patients has become as easy as brewing a cup of coffee.

To this day, Guo continues to revise products, creating new formulas and new methods for Western lifestyles. Life Rising's research institute, clinic, and herbal manufacturing company in China all continue to create quality products for modern needs.[1]

He was not just a Chinese medicine practitioner; he was actually a MD doctor and a surgeon. I am so happy I decided to go there and see what he had to say. It took only two weeks before I started feeling better. We are still working together, taking my health ahead one step at the time. We have also had multiple conversations in which Dr. Guo explained me the entire workings behind Chinese medicine.

### IS IT RIGHT FOR YOU?

I truly believe you should get familiar with this methodology, as it as it

---

1. Used with permission. For more information, go to http://www.liferising.com/about/guo.html

might really work for you. It certainly made huge difference in my life. As Dr. Guo explains on his website (See Appendix II), in general, TCM is an ancient discipline, going back more than 3000 years. It focuses on acupuncture and herbal remedies, but also includes diet, exercise, and even psychological and emotional issues. Its goal is to restore the body to its natural healthy state; not to "treat illnesses" as such.

What makes TCM different from Western medicine is that it is holistic. In other words, it looks at the connections between a person's health, lifestyle, environment, and personality. In TCM, health is a result of balance in the body and "illness" is the result of imbalance. Each organ has a specific function, not just as in Western medicine, but in Qi, or life force energy. TCM relies heavily on observation of subtle signs in the patient, such as my paleness and color or my tongue.

As my master Dr. Guo says, "Every illness is a struggle within the body between the forces of the illness or disease pathogens, and the resources and abilities of the body to fight them off. The direction of this struggle determines the recovery of the individual. To correct imbalances that underlie various conditions, TCM aims to restore the original, natural balance of the body's internal functions."

## YOUR CHOICE

It is really entirely up to you, which medicinal path you take, or maybe you will combine both, as I did. It would be sad if someone would try to convince you to go with conventional medicine just for financial benefits. As in any area of our lives, I believe in cooperation and dialog between all parties involved.

Since the medical community has not yet found a cure for endometriosis, I believe that your decision of leaning towards remedies you feel will help you should be highly respected. If something works for you, just go with it.

---

1. Used with permission. For more information, go to http://www.liferising.com/about/guo.html

I was told hormones would work for me, but they did not; they suppressed pain but caused other problems. I knew I could not tell my doctor that I was going with my own way of healing; he would not understand, he would feel insulted and he would not feel responsible for my well-being.

I have helped many women with their pain, fatigue and other symptoms. There is nothing more rewarding to me to replace the tears with a nice bright smile. Nothing feels better than bringing comfort to someone who is desperate to find the quality of life that endometriosis has stolen.

Listen to your body and the smallest signal it sends you, because it has lots to say. As Frank Navarti says, "Often as we travel, we come across several obstacles in our lives or crossroads that present to us a variety of direction to take. There is no right or wrong direction if we listen to our intuition and to our heart."

# CHAPTER 11 | Life with Endometriosis

I wish I could tell you something different, but currently, there is no cure for endometriosis. Suggesting specific treatment for endometriosis is difficult, due to the individual make up of each woman. You and your physician need to discuss your goals and the benefits and risks of the treatment options to determine which is best for you. The type of treatment you choose depends on your age, disease, symptoms, and whether you want to have children. While treatment may relieve your pain for a while and enable you to get pregnant, your symptoms may come back after treatment. As much as we wish there were a cure, unfortunately, claims of cures are absolutely untrue. Surgery does not cure endometriosis; lasers do not cure endometriosis; pregnancy does not cure endometriosis; hysterectomy does not cure endometriosis; menopause does not cure endometriosis; birth control pills do not cure endometriosis; dietary changes do not cure endometriosis.

There is no cure for endometriosis.

However, there is life after the diagnosis.

## NO DAY THE SAME

No two days are the same with endometriosis. Sometimes I am well and I can achieve a lot, and some days I struggle to walk. It is the random element of this disease that proves to be one of the biggest frustrations. I do not know how much energy I will have until I open my eyes. Some only feel pain for a few days a month; some are in pain all the time. It is an extremely varied illness.

Also confusing is the fact that many women with endometriosis never experience any symptoms at all. They only find out something is wrong when trying to have a child.

## THE EXHAUSTION OF ILLNESS

Any long-term illness is tiring. A relatively normal day of activity requires a lot of hard work and forward planning on the part of the person that is suffering. Chronic fatigue is one of the frequently overlooked symptoms of endometriosis, but is also one of the most common, and among the trickiest to manage alongside the pain. When you are pain-filled, your stress levels elevate so that it becomes harder to think, form sentences, to remember things, or perform actions were even once easy, like speaking calmly. Like our illness, life fluctuates from day to day, depending on how much we have to do, how much pain we are in, and how much energy we have.

Despite the confusion and misinformation continuing to surround the disease, the profound, agonizing pain caused by endometriosis is actually treatable, and in many cases quite successfully.

Unfortunately, due to a lack of societal and medical community awareness, women are frequently directed to "manage" their discomfort for years with powerful painkillers and hormones, but these only mask symptoms of the condition. What's more, many patients are incorrectly informed by their doctors and treated for symptoms but not the disease itself, which consequently causes a long delay in effective treatment. This dangerous result has led to many "hit or miss" surgeries and thousands of unnecessary hysterectomies. Laparoscopic Excision Surgery is an effective, organ-sparing option; ideally performed by experienced, specialized surgeons with dedicated, multidisciplinary medical teams.

I have emphasized repeatedly that endometriosis is a common, yet poorly understood disease that can strike women of any socioeconomic class, age, or race. The disease can affect nearly every aspect of a woman's life - her ability to work, her ability to reproduce, and her relationships with her mate, her child, and everyone around her.

## ON THE FRONT LINES

We women with endometriosis command the front lines. In our daily lives we are bosses, teachers, and police officers; we are important members of a constantly moving, ever-present society. We must be on duty 24/7, yet often pain gets in our way. And yet, when we dare ask for reinforcements, we are pegged "quitters," or worse, the daily battle we fight is "all in our heads."

Doctors shrug off our pain and downplay the war waging in our pelvises. They toss a new strategy to keep the battle going - antidepressants, other drugs, the list is endless. Nevertheless, until a covert mission (i.e. a laparoscopy) is ordered, doctors will not invest in the battle. In addition, getting a doctor to sign off on that mission can be near impossible – at least until you have exhausted their mini attacks without success.

Some will say that the endometriosis war is a series of hellish battles. And I would agree. There is the daily battle of depression, isolation, and anguish, all physical symptoms that are beyond physical understanding. There is the ongoing battle to get a diagnosis. Navigating the healthcare system is a daunting task. Finally there is the battle of knowing. Its wounds are denial (even if you've been searching for this answer, it's normal to question the diagnosis), anger (your body has failed you; doctors may have taken years to diagnose you or are suggesting a treatment you're not comfortable with; or they believe you're infertile), bargaining (this one applies especially to endometriosis patients who experience infertility), depression, and finally acceptance.

## WE MUST PERSEVERE

Regardless of where we are in the war, one thing is certain: we must persevere. We must press for further research and back scientific endeavors searching for a cure. We must write our political figures and insist on protective legislation. We must stand firm and say NO to doctors when we feel uncomfortable about a drug or surgical treatment. We must feel empowered.

## SISTERS IN THE BATTLE

I personally believe that the greatest asset doctors and researchers have is all the women in the world who have even the smallest symptoms of endometriosis.

We are very important and valuable. We are needed!

We are even more important when we talk and share and open up. It is ok to talk about endometriosis, but it's not ok to go alone through the Death Valley with no hope of drop of rain.

It's unbelievably important to share your story. Would you take it more seriously if I tell you that your story can rescue one life? Would you feel good if you were the reason why other women know more? I can't emphasize enough the importance of sharing and power of creating community, collaboration, and interexchange. I don't know of any successful company, accomplishment, or single individual who is solely responsible for success.

I believe sharing good things multiplies them; sharing pain and sorrow divides it and makes it lesser. Maybe not necessarily physically in our cases, but it gives us feeling of not being lonely or abandoned in these complex situations. Hence I will again encourage you to tell your story. Tell it no matter how painful it may be. It may be a story which may contribute to save one more soul.

I am grateful for anyone who shared their story with me. Each story was individual, each one of them was special, and each one of them was moving. I want you to remember that the more we uncover the more evidence we deliver.

I would love you to join me in a journey of looking for those who are alone and scared to get out and name this "something" eating them alive. I think we owe them the ability to regain their quality of life.

I have now shared with you all that I currently know about the disease of endometriosis. While I do not know you personally, I feel like you are my sisters. And as sisters, we will continue to battle this dreaded disease until a cure can be found. This is OUR fight. Learning each other's stories, talking about our struggles, acknowledging our pain and sharing our lives is the way to finally realize that we are never alone.

Self-healing and self-love are the true obstacles we face in our journey through life. Endometriosis has certainly taught me so much about myself, my body and how life can really be a test of courage and self-love. It is because of endometriosis that I can honestly say that I love you, and I am here for you, should you need to contact me.

## MY LIFE

Finally, I want to encourage you by sharing one of my mornings with you. I hope you can identify with my feelings and realize that no matter how bad you feel right now, you can still have an amazing life!

*I wake up. I open my eyes, not sure what time it is just yet. I look through half-closed eyes and see that it's a cloudy, cloudy morning.*

*Ehh....*

*Weekend it is, so I don't have to get up. I can stay in bed, cover myself with my soft comfy blanket, and pretend I haven't woken up yet.*

*Naaah...*

I decide to get up. I leave my warm bed, put my robe on and go downstairs. It's still cloudy as I fix a warm cup of coffee. I cup it in my hands and look out at the hazy morning. I could go for a run I think. For a moment, I waver, undecided, then I put down my coffee cup, go back upstairs and get dressed in my running clothes.

As I step outside, the cool morning air hits my face and I am tempted to go back inside. But I don't.

I begin to run, slow at first, but then picking up speed. I run over a small hill and all of a sudden, I don't see the clouds anymore and I don't feel the cold.

I feel well, energized, refreshed, and encouraged. My lungs open and I take in the fresh air of a brand-new day. I laugh at myself for thinking I might not go on this run. Why would I give up something like this just because it's Saturday morning? We never say, "Oh I won't bother eating today because it's Saturday."

I keep running. I run past a man getting his morning paper. I run past another woman jogging with her dog. I don't think of anything. I just breathe. I just relax. I just enjoy.

All of a sudden, a ray of sunshine breaks through the clouds and my spirits lift even higher. I know it's going to be an amazing day!

I get home, a little sweaty, but feeling like I can do anything! I reward myself with juice made from green apples, carrots, celery, and pears. As I drink the life-giving nutrients, I feel strong, I feel confident, I feel ready for any challenge.

I may have endometriosis, but that doesn't mean that my life is over. It is just the beginning.

Together we can become all that we are meant to be.

With hope for a bright future for you!

Ania

# CHAPTER 12

## *EndoPositive*™ *International*
### A Global Community is Born

EndoPositive.org

When you are sick all you want is to be healthy, but when you are healthy you want it all. They tell you to dream big and to shoot for the stars and they tell you that you can have all you want if you set your mind to it, but is it really so?

I believe! But the first and most important thing is your ultimate well being, without it there is no dreams as health is the only one that matters.

A woman's health is more than just the health of one individual, it is far beyond. When you pay attention to the trends of women's empowerment in business, families, the beauty industry and when you analyze consumerism you see an enormous impact of females everywhere in the world. From family, beauty,

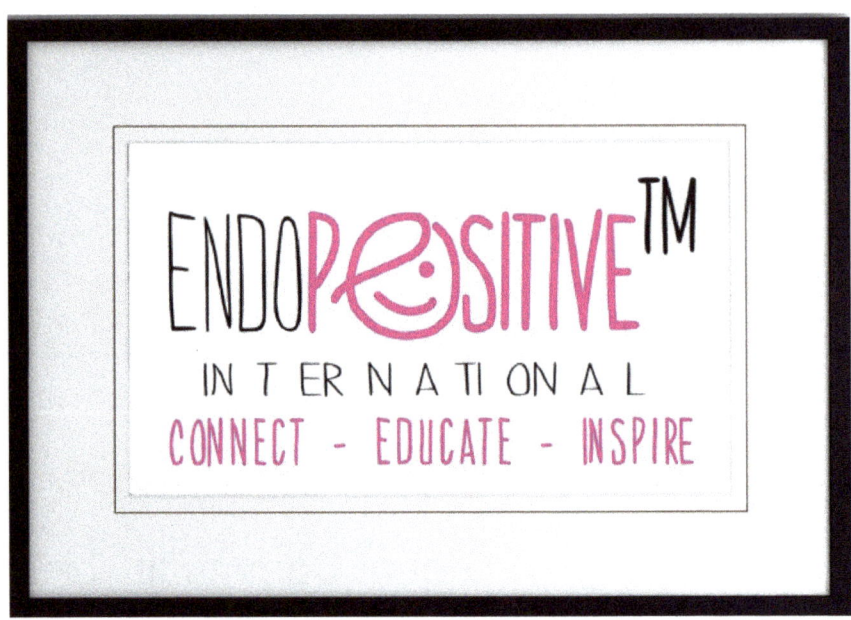

health, fashion to business, politics and justice. Women cover it all. Despite their state of health they push themselves to fulfill their role properly.

Women' bodies are all together and partially exposed and used for various purposes. Depending on the culture in some way or another whether it is her breast, legs or her smile it is either for sale, to admire or to critique.

Perhaps you do not realize and for sure you should give it a thought that very often behind this beautiful face and smile there is a lot of pain, tears and sorrow. To keep this smile up they are served pain killers, drugs, antidepressant and numerous surgeries. They are no longer treated as souls but rather as a property which serves purposes of some sort.

We pay attention to animal cruelty and we raise money to make sure they have homes, we pay attention to homeless people and we put roof over their heads. And we take credit for it while meantime we enjoy beautiful faces and don't even bother to wonder what is backstage as the facade is too beautiful and we are blown away.

Let's move on further, when you are no longer a Goddess and it is time for you to conceive and you have trouble to so you are served remedies that miraculously will let you deliver to the world an heir. When things are good, it's all good, but what happens when you deliver a child who is sick, misshaped and nobody knows why? No one will want to admit that perhaps the amount of pharmaceuticals a women consumed may have caused side effects and now we need to raise more money for the mother and for the baby and for the medical industry to find out what is it that it is born as there are only 6 cases like this in the world! What a circle? I should rather say what a vicious circle?!

Don't you think it needs to stop? Don't you think someone has to? If we will not stop it now, we are about to give a birth to totally handicap generation! Question is who will take care of them when we will be old. So far without anyone interfering this is a recipe for self distraction.

I believe that death is a spiritual problem not medical so we cannot stop it, however we may stop the unconscious, blind and thoughtless worship to the so called science of the medical world. We have to stop taking for granted what we are told or made to believe. We need to develop an extra sense of alertness of why we are told things and ask; where are we going next?

When you are in pain or when you suffer from debilitating illness it is very hard to keep your cool and not to lose it or it is very hard nearly impossible to turn on your common sense and it is totally impossible when you are drugged and thinking is not even an option.

In the process of observing all of this EndoPositive International™ was born. It is a worldwide educational organization whose goal is to provide connection, community and support for women globally to help with prevention and pre-emptively promote wellness. In fact, at EndoPositive International™ our tag line is: connect, educate, inspire. But it's much more than just a fun sounding tagline it's something thousands of women experience daily with their peers from around the globe.

We work together with many doctors from all medical modalities that are hand-picked and true to their core values. We believe that education will give you the power and right to make the right choices for you and your loved ones.

It is very easy to get lost in today's world of information overflow. It is very confusing on who is really an expert and why would they call themselves so. We are coming here to teach you how to recognize all of these and how to pick what has true value.

EPI is an interactive education where you can gain all the information and create a complete library of wellness. It is education for everyone no exception. Parents, children, siblings, businesses, employers, husbands, partners and doctors. We are here for those who are lucky and are healthy but they want to deepen their knowledge on health and health industry. These members will be able to prevent from getting into pitfalls of medical industry. On the other hand these who are on the way there or even deep there will be able to gain support of how to change the route and get on the right truck. We offer psychological support for every individual, giving you the support you need to find stability and get better.

EPI is a safe community where women can get connection, content and digital education. Our interest is not the object but the subject. You are the most important. You need to know what you do and what you consume and you deserve to know what will happen to you after you do so. We are too advanced in science to tell you: maybe this will be a solution. We are pretty much able to predict the consequences.

As a patient you should know all, and nothing should be confidential if it is safe right? We are working with doctors from every modality that are highly qualified to contribute to your well being. Gaining knowledge is a choice and not gaining it is taking a chance. Now you can decide.

A portion of the proceeds from the sale of each book will go to support the ongoing efforts and work of EndoPositive.org because I believe so strongly in what we are doing here. When you go to AniaLive.com you can easily purchase my book for yourself and a friend.

---

[19] http://www.mayoclinic.org/diseases-conditions/endometriosis/basics/treatment/con-20013968

# APPENDIX III: Alternative Treatments

Various types of alternative/natural treatments are available for endometriosis. Some of these include:

- Reduce exposure to toxic chemical such as dioxin by cutting back on dairy and red meat.
- Eat more vegetables that contain flavones, the enzyme that converts androgens to estrogens. Good sources are celery, broccoli, cauliflower, and kale.
- Include Omega-3 Fatty acids found in fish like salmon

and mackerel or in fish oil capsules as part of your diet.
- Reduce stress. While stress doesn't cause endometriosis, it can make dealing with it more difficult.
- Consult a homeopathy or naturopathy for supplement suggestions such as B vitamins and magnesium.
- Try Traditional Chinese Medicine including herbs and acupuncture.
- Manage your diet by avoiding fatty foods, sugar, and caffeine.
- Add gentle exercise such as walking, swimming, or yoga to help with both fitness and stress management.
- Get regular massages to help control pain and reduce tension.

# APPENDIX IV | *Eating with Endo*

As I said earlier, changing my diet was an essential part of my recovery. I firmly believe that food is the best medicine. Even if you don't have a "cure," you will feel so much better and be able to deal with the stresses of endometriosis when your body is well fed and well nourished.

When I was a kid I hated vegetables! Just thinking of eating salad made my face sour. I so much preferred meat and sausage from boring veggies. I gave my parents, who tried to make sure I am getting all the nutrients I needed, a very hard time!

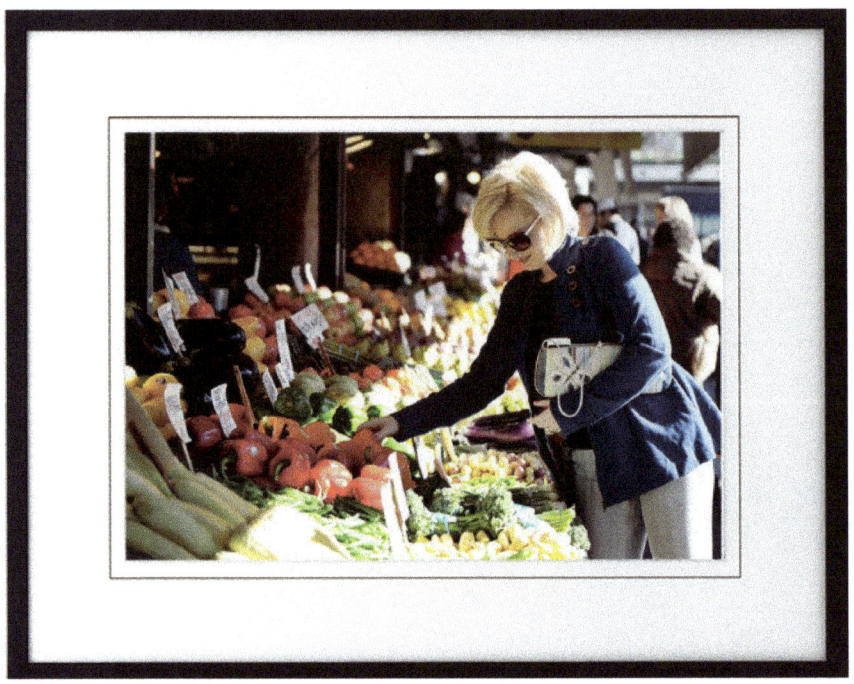

Today I look back and I realize these were best veggies I could have consumed! They came straight from my grandpa's garden. I couldn't get anything more organic then this!

When dealing with endometriosis, you should eat organic as often as possible, because the pesticide residue found on many non-organic food items may also increase estrogens in your body.

When you are shopping for fruits, try to look for local produce for two reasons. First most of the time it will be so much more likely to be really organic. Second you will be supporting your local business. I am very sentimental about it as I remember my grandfather sharing his natural goods with others. Just thinking of it makes me have nice warm memories.

Being conscious of eating fruits and veggies is extremely important for your health. In my childhood, access to tropical fruits was very limited and once we had them, consuming them became a special occasion. This is why today I don't take them for granted and I hope you don't either.

Besides eating more fruits and vegetables, other suggestions include:

- Avoid wheat because wheat feeds Candida growth and many women with endometriosis suffer from Candida overgrowth.
- Cut out or reduce red meat and dairy, which are known to increase prostaglandins, the chemicals that produce pain signals in the body. Natural yogurt (not the commercial sweet flavored yogurts) is the exception to the no-dairy rule because it contains bacteria that can help with your digestion and to combat Candida overgrowth.
- Reduce or eliminate sugar. Sugar feeds Candida and increases painful inflammation.
- Reduce or eliminate caffeine found in coffee, tea, and soft drinks.
- Increase consumption of "good oils" meaning natural, unrefined cold-pressed oils such as safflower, walnut, flax seed, and coconut.
- Eat more whole grains such as oatmeal, brown rice, barley, quinoa, and spelt. Avoid GMO modified corn and wheat products.
- Increase your intake of beans, colorful fruits like red berries and apples, garlic, cauliflower, broccoli, carrots, beets, and green vegetables.
- Eat organic vegetarian-fed chicken and organic fish. If you must eat red meat make sure it is organic.
- Add sea salt to your food in place of table salt. Sea sale provides natural iodine and other minerals that modern diets often lack.

So what are some of my favorite foods?

Apples are at the top of my list. There are so many benefits of eating apples from regulating your blood sugar and preventing cardiovascular disease to anti-cancer benefits to being great antioxidants and many more.

When you go shopping for apples don't look for the ones that are perfectly shaped and shiny from waxing. Rather look for those that are not so pretty; they will have fewer chemicals. I do not recall apples in my grandpa's orchard that were all same in shape. But I remember they were so juicy and sweet!

*Celery* perhaps won't be your choice and maybe not first on your list, but it definitely is one of the very valuable veggies and one of my favorites. It's an ideal anti-inflammatory remedy. I was never crazy about celery and its very intense taste but I've learned to appreciate it. I am sure oxidative stress and cancer ring the bell, and if so - think celery! You can't go wrong.

*Pineapple* is such a Hawaiian fruit. Are you thinking Pina colada? I do to! I don't believe I have to convince anyone why we should eat pineapple. It's sweet, juicy, refreshing. It's giving you just this warm tropical feeling of sitting on the beach and sipping its juice. But believe me; it's not just tasty it's also very healthy!

*Carrots* are a versatile veggie. As a child I was not that friendly with them. I changed my mind and we became real good friends. They are not only healthy for your body, but also beneficial for your eyes and skin. They are tasty alone, in a cake, in a juice, and even rabbits love them!

# APPENDIX V | The Sweet Life

I love chocolate! Just looking at this word makes me smell its fragrance and I smile. Unfortunately, I had to cut off all the refined sugars and sweets in general and I am glad I did. However I found my own desserts that are organic, healthy, and actually good for you.

Here are few of my secrets, which with illustrations by Ewaso, my great friend and supporter.

# Strawberry Delight

You will need:
- 2 cups fresh strawberries
- ¼ cup frozen pineapple
- ¼ cup almond milk
- 1 tbs agave syrup. If you feel like you would like it even sweeter, you may add one tbs of agave syrup and blend it together.
- 1 or 2 peppermint leaves

Blend strawberries (room temperature)
Pour blended mousse in a nice tall glass dish.
Pour almond milk into a blender, add frozen pineapples, and blend together.
Once done, pour it slowly over your strawberry mousse.
Top it with peppermint leaves for a nice fresh scent and refreshment.
That simple? Yes! Enjoy.

# Energy Bars

You will need:
- 1 cup of dates pitted
- 1 cup of Turkish figs
- 1 cup of fresh almonds
- 2 tbs raw unsweetened cacao
- 1 ripe kiwi
- 1 tbs vanilla extract
- Pinch of Himalayan salt
- Dates, figs, and almonds

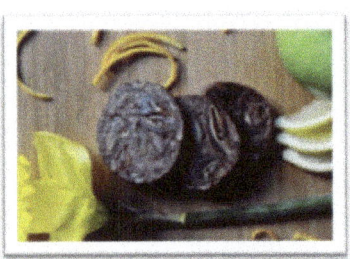

Cut dates and figs in small pieces or cubes and place it in a glass bowl. Grind almonds in a blender until fine. Your almonds need to become your flour.

> Add cacao, vanilla extract and pinch of Himalayan salt.
> Peel your kiwi and smash it to puree.

Knead all the ingredients together until they are blended into a ball. Form the ball into a round long shape, so that later you may cut it in thin medallions. Wrap it in a plastic foil and place in a freezer. You may store it there for about two weeks and have it handy for whenever you will crave for it.

It is a great desert when you are tired and need energy or after your workout. One thin piece is plenty. You will find this out very quickly.

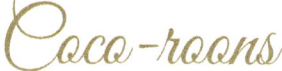

## Coco-roons

- 2 cups of shredded coconut
- 1 cup of fresh almonds
- ½ cup of maple syrup
- 2 tbs cacao
- Pinch of Himalayan salt
- 1 tbs vanilla extract

Grind 1 cup coconut and almonds into flour. Place the flour and the rest of coconuts into a bowl. Add maple syrup, cacao, salt, and vanilla extract.

Knead all together and form small balls. You need to make them really tight.

At the end, you may deep them into shredded coconut for a nice fluffy look.

# APPENDIX VI | The Juicy Life

One of the most famous writers in Poland wrote an epigram on health. He said that unfortunately we mostly cherish our health after we have already lost it. True or not there is something about to his saying. We tend to take things for granted and we think we are untouchable.

On the other hand, there is also another group of individuals who are very conscious and they do all they can to prevent their well-being from deteriorating before it's too late.

I am not certain to which group you belong but I hope that you begin to take steps right now either to regain your health or to keep from losing it.

One of the best ways I know is to juice. Even though my parents and grandparents tried to make eating fruits and vegetables a priority, I wish back then they had known about juicing. Since I can't get the time back, I now juice every day and I encourage you to do the same.

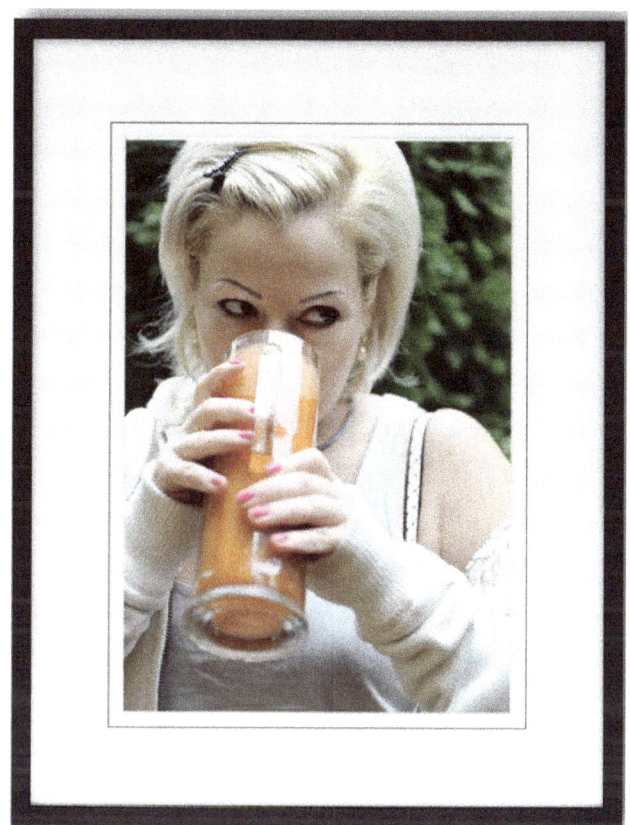

For all the following juices, wash the fruits and vegetables thoroughly to get rid of pesticides and chemicals. It isn't necessary to peel them as long as you wash them. (The exception is citrus fruits like lemons or limes. They need to be peeled before juicing). Cut into chunks that will fit into your blender and remove any seeds or pits.

## Pineapple Carrot Juice

You will need:

- 5 large carrots
- 1 large green apple
- 1/4 pineapple
- 4 stalks of celery

## Apple Celery Juice

- 2 green apples, halved
- 4 stalks celery, leaves removed
- 1 cucumber
- 6 leaves kale
- 1/2 lemon, peeled
- 1 (1 inch) piece fresh ginger

## Cucumber Refresher

- 2 cucumbers
- 1 fresh lime or lemon (peel first)
  Juice the cucumbers and lime or lemon, then add
- 1 to 2 tsp agave syrup & 1 cup fresh water

## Apple Beet Combo

- 1 small beet (or half of a large one)
- 2 carrots
- 1 apple
- 2 to 3 leaves of kale

# APPENDIX VII | Restaurants

Eating out can be a challenge while being on a diet, struggling with weight, or suffering from health condition and being limited with what you can or cannot eat.

That very often becomes THE reason why we prefer to stay home and we start to isolate ourselves. Sadly, doing so can lead to much deeper issues. So right now I just want to talk about eating out.

No one likes to be odd. I am not talking about being different, original, or unique. I am referring to someone who is particularly picky about a place to eat, what food to eat, what time to eat and so forth. Even though such demands may come from reasons other than just being capricious, being the center of attention is not exactly what I would be looking for.

Going out with bunch of people who are not your friends but maybe potential clients or business partners is not easy when you have to take their preferences under consideration before yours.

I have been in such situations numerous times, and fortunately, I found my way around these. Since I am mostly vegetarian and going vegan on occasion, it is not always easy to find foods that will suit my liking. Taking under consideration the "meaty" tastes of others, I need to improve my communication with the wait staff... so far so good!

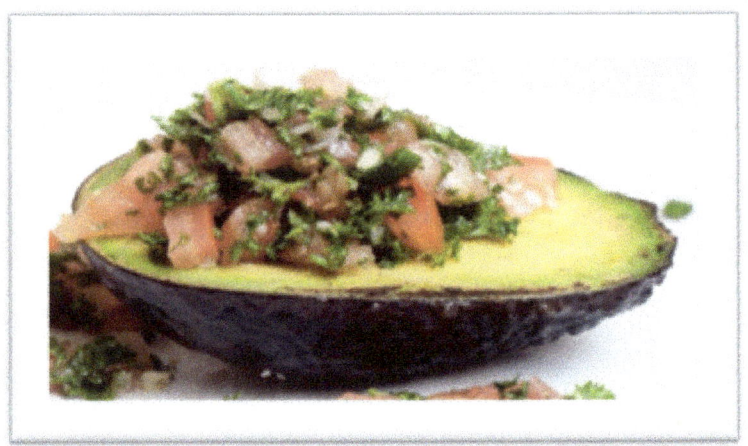

Of course, I don't tell everyone why I make my food choices; that would prolong each meeting and gathering for ages! And frankly, who cares why you are weird!

There is no need to do tell everyone, so you can keep your secret for yourself. While everybody else is sitting in a steak restaurant and debating how they want their meat cooked, I am browsing through salads and veggie sides. Restaurants always have these on a menu. I am always the first one who makes up her mind my choice of a meal. So from being supposedly moody, I am the first one ready!

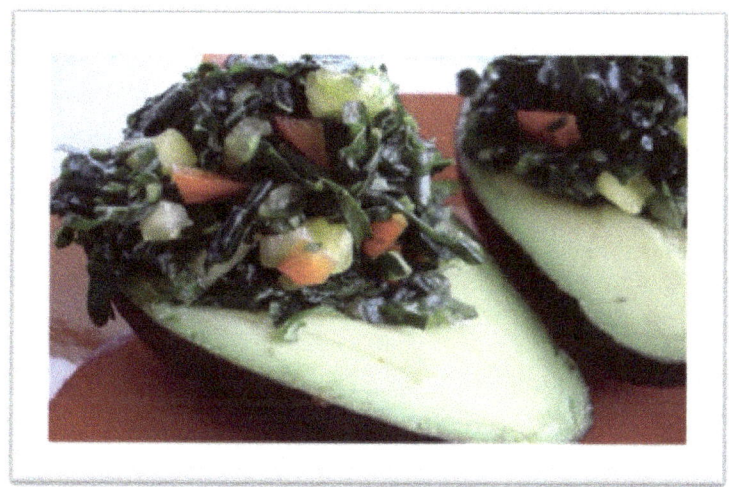

On the other hand, if there is nothing on a menu I could eat without paying for it later due to some kind of pain, I approach the staff kindly and ask for an avocado. Most often, they have these in stock and I love this fruit. It is filling, very high in nutrients, and makes for a great meal.

Adding salt, pepper, and lemon will do it for me. However, many times I have been in a restaurant where the waitress brought it to me nicely prepared with some salsa or steamed veggies - what a nice surprise! I don't know if you are an avocado lover, but if not, perhaps this is the way to start. It's healthy food for your soul and brain.

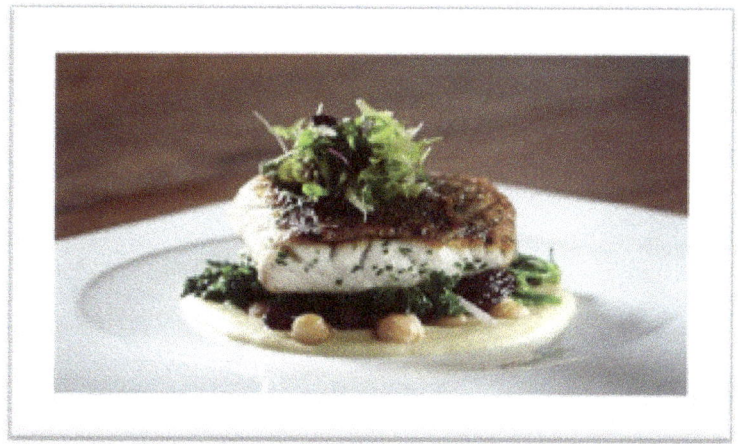

I was born a meat eater, with sausage in one hand and sausage in another. But suffering with endometriosis caused me to make a major shift that was not that easy. How could I ever live without meat? Yet I didn't have much choice if I wanted to start feeling better. My body was constantly tired, and eating meat and digesting it was taking too much of my energy! Fish came from heaven - light, delicate, and very filling. Since most of the restaurants serve fish, it makes my life very easy and my belly very happy!

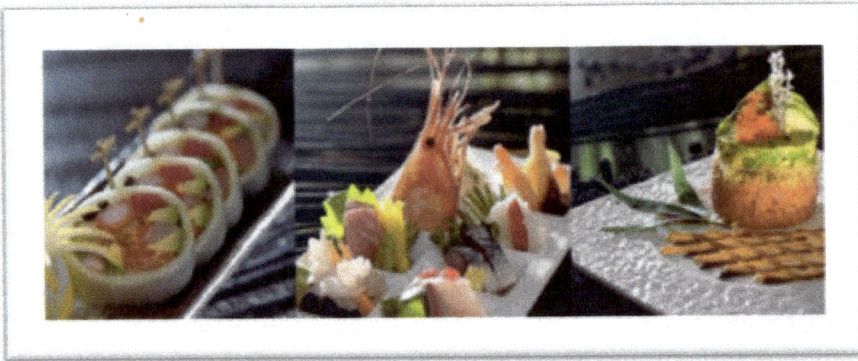

And of course I love sushi! Anytime, anywhere but the best I have ever had was in California. Now that I live here, it's a bonus!

Unfortunately, many of my friends don't like it because it is raw. Hence, when I get a chance to go with people who choose it, I take advantage. Good sushi places always have veggie rolls and delicious seaweed salad. Sushi is a good, wholesome, and light food.

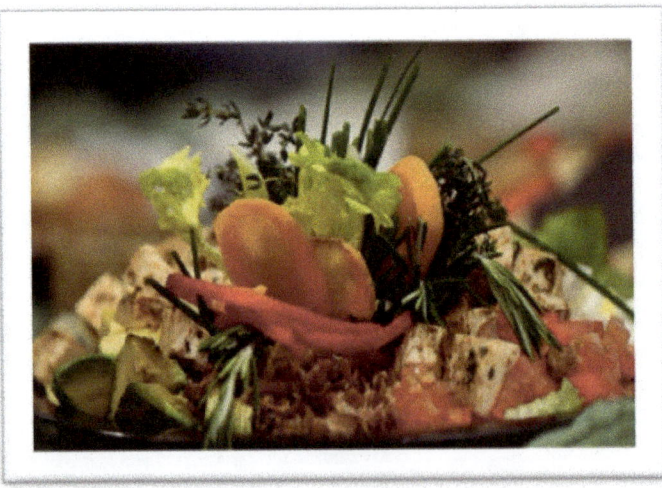

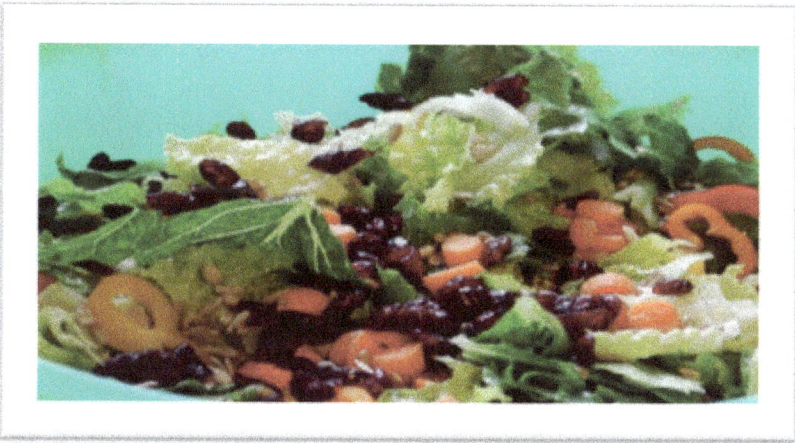

Salads of course! They don't have to be boring. Again, even there is nothing on menu you are crazy about, or salads seem poor and boring, you may certainly ask for add-ons. I cannot recall one time someone at a restaurant ever turned my request down.

I need to add one very important thing. Maybe you know this already, but if not, DO NOT EAT Iceberg lettuce. I know it's juicy and very crunchy, and has a great texture; unfortunately, it is manufactured and not organic in any shape or form. Instead, romaine lettuce, mixed greens, arugula, and other natural greens are all good, healthy, and available in any restaurant.

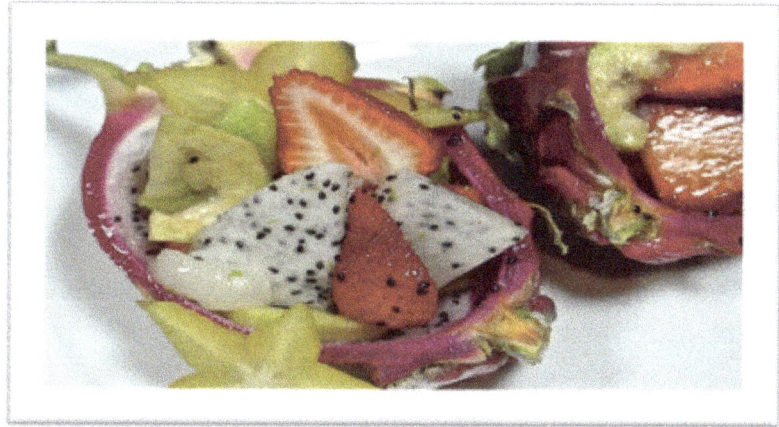

Desert time is tempting and challenging. But whether or not you have endometriosis, or you are perfectly healthy, I am sure you are watching your figure. For some reason, while going out for dinner we forget about fruit platters as desert; perhaps we think of them as best served with breakfast or lunch. Let this serve as a sweet reminder about the many juicy, colorful, and yummy fruit combinations that will complement your meal. Dragon fruit, star fruit, kiwi… if you haven't tried these, don't wait! Treat yourself right away.

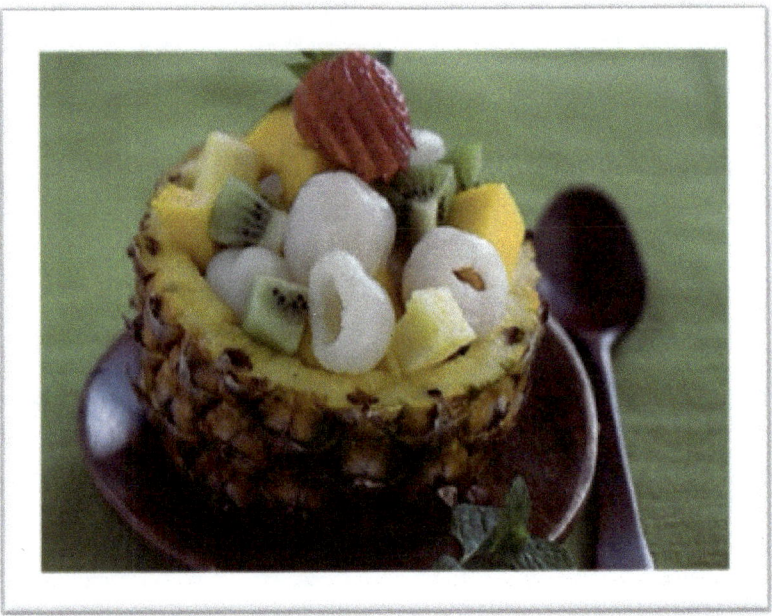

I hope you will find this advice helpful, and you will no longer stay home because eating out was not fun until now. You do not need to isolate yourself just because your food choices are different. You also do not need to eat things that will make you sick or cause you pain.

Staying positive and knowing people will work with you should encourage you greatly. The weekend is just ahead; make plans and enjoy! Keep me posted about what you're up to on social media AniaLive.com and I will follow you back!

A portion of the proceeds from the sale of each book will go to support the ongoing efforts and work of EndoPositive.org because I believe so strongly in what we are doing here. When you go to AniaLive.com you can easily purchase my book for yourself and a friend.

I really do hope to meet you in person soon. Until we do you can reach me on both of the above Websites and you can share your story with me and thousands of other Endo Sisters around the globe and YOUR STORY can inspire others to LIVE WELL WITH ENDOMETRIOSIS! Thank you for taking time to read my story. Feel free to share it with other and if we ever get to actual meet in person, I'd love that!

*Ania G*

We'll see you on the inside! The world is waiting to hear YOUR story at EndoPositive.org

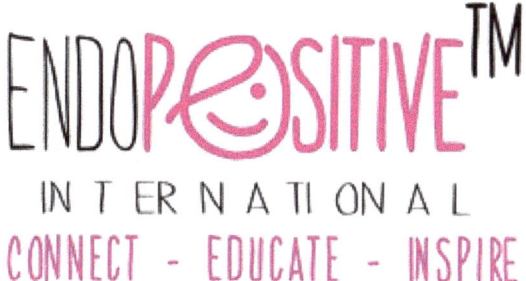

www.ingramcontent.com/pod-product-compliance
Lightning Source LLC
LaVergne TN
LVHW051225070526
838200LV00057B/4603